You Don't Know What You Don't Know

The Health and Safety Guide
For
College Students
(and All Students of Life)

ISBN-10: 1451577621
EAN-13: 9781451577624

You Don't Know What You Don't Know

The Health and Safety Guide
For
College Students
(and All Students of Life)

William Bhaskar, MD
Philip Bhaskar, DMD

"The wisest mind has something yet to learn."
George Santayana   1863-1952

TERMS AND CONDITIONS
<u>READ CAREFULLY BEFORE USING THIS BOOK</u>

Dedication

To our parents, who taught us first.
To our professors, who taught us skills.
To our children, who teach us still.

The Website

www.ydkWydk.com

"Nothing endures but change."
Heraclitus   540 BC-480 BC

It is estimated that clinical medical knowledge doubles every seven years, and that the sum of all human knowledge doubles yearly. This explosion of wisdom enhances and enriches our lives and health, yet staying current is a challenge. Therefore, the primary goal of the website is to be a portal to legitimate and credible medical references, advances and breakthroughs. The internet is unsurpassed for education, and the website will enhance the book with in-depth discussions and media illustrations. Links to references, sources and innovative products, as well as downloads of forms and checklists, will be available.

"When I was a boy of fourteen, my father was so ignorant I could hardly stand to have the old man around. But when I got to be twenty-one, I was astonished by how much he'd learned in seven years."

Attributed to Mark Twain   1835-1910

Authors' Note

The book began as a labor of love for our sons and daughters, nieces and nephews, as they reached adulthood and left for college. It was originally intended to be a guide to basic health and safety, not much more than a small, handy manual covering salient and critical issues, similar to the "peripheral brain" we carried in our doctor's coats during clinical training. However, as we researched topics and listened to feedback, we gradually expanded the scope of the manual to include things that we always did for them and they had yet to do for themselves, such as book airline travel or deal with the aftermath of an automobile accident. We have drawn from our years of surgical training, life experience and scientific observation in an attempt to spare them the pain of repeating our, and others', mistakes and misfortunes. We have published this book to share this information with all college students and other students of life in the hope that we can all learn from each other.

"I don't think much of a man who is not wiser today than he was yesterday."

Abraham Lincoln 1809-1865

Introduction

The authors believe that medical education and knowledge are crucial to health, wellness and longevity. Our goal is to educate and empower patients to understand how their bodies function and to take steps to maintain and improve their health continually through life. To that end, we have tried to present the major health and wellness issues that confront young adults through middle age.

The scope of this book is immense and wide-ranging. Our intent was to cover as many crucial topics as possible, minimize medical jargon, and still keep the book small and handy. The two authoritative medical texts, *Harrison's Principles of Internal Medicine* and *Schwartz's Principles of Surgery* are huge, heavy tomes of almost five thousand pages. The constraints of size, readability and range create certain unavoidable limitations that the reader must understand and accept.

In medicine, treatment is tailored to the unique patient and situation. Medical treatment for a 21 year old athlete is different from a 62 year old diabetic with heart disease, even if they both present with the same symptom of headache. Even the same patient will have different needs at different stages of life. It is incumbent upon the reader to understand that this text is not medical diagnosis or treatment, but rather a broad overview of health topics from which to begin a lifelong study of their own health and medicine. We advise that the reader keep abreast of advances in health and nutrition, and follow advancements in the treatment of their specific illness or condition.

Medical knowledge and technology changes and evolves constantly. Every day new studies and findings change the way physicians diagnose and treat disease. The reader is encouraged to seek authoritative reference sources such as www.webMD.com , www.nih.gov , www.cdc.gov or www.mayoclinic.com for definitive and peer reviewed overviews and treatment options.

Contents

PERSONAL SAFETY

MOTOR VEHICLE SAFETY

TRAVEL SAFETY

KEYS TO SUCCESS

FINAL THOUGHTS

REFERENCES AND RESOURCES 275

INDEX 281

ABOUT THE AUTHORS 288

FUNDAMENTALS

The Surgeon's Perspective

As the authors are both doctors, our outlook is colored by our training and our experience. One trained as a plastic and reconstructive surgeon and the other as an oral and maxillofacial surgeon, both acquiring analytical thought processes that govern our practices and lives. The dominant tenet that guides us is a principle used by diagnosticians in examining patients:

If it looks like a duck,

If it walks like a duck,

If it quacks like a duck,

It is probably a duck.

If you are assessing a patient in extremis, and you begin the workup suspecting the most arcane and rare illness, he will surely expire before you work through to the most common and likely diagnosis. Common things are common.

The other concern that all surgeons face is risk. With every procedure, there is risk and reward. The surgeon is trained to assess risk, understand potential complications, and be able to avoid or treat them. We expect the best outcome, yet prepare for the worst. This may seem obvious, but the implications are far reaching. This book was written with that mindset.

We approach each challenge, and life in general, by assessing the risks. What that means in regards to this book is that we have given priority to high incidence events and issues. There is no discussion of obscure brain tumors here because, thankfully, they are rare. We will discuss motor vehicle accidents because, tragically, almost half of the readers of this book will be involved in one in their lifetime. We have attempted to address the major risks that face adults in modern life, clearly and concisely.

Pearls of Wisdom

Pearls are a traditional teaching technique in medical, dental and surgical education. When the young doctor is inundated with an overwhelming deluge of scientific information, identifying the key, critical facts helps immensely. Success in life is about wise choices and wise choices require knowledge. For example, if 85% of dog bites come from Rottweilers or pit bulls, one might be prudent knowing what those breeds look like. The text is formatted in a manner to emphasize these pearls. It is our sincere hope that this knowledge will help keep the reader healthy and safe in our vast and wonderful but sometimes dangerous world.

The Scientific Method

The cock crows at dawn, but he doesn't raise the sun.

Thinkers since Aristotle have explored the mysteries of the physical universe using the scientific method. Scholars search for the *cause and effect* relationship behind natural phenomena. This process is the basis of all scientific advancement.

Facts alone can be deceptive. Facts can be twisted to support a false hypothesis, or interpreted incorrectly. Example: 85% of shark attacks occur in waist deep water. But what does that mean? That 85% of sharks live in shallow water? That sharks come to shallow water to feed? That sharks breed in shallow water, therefore they are more aggressive? That you have an 85% chance of being bitten in shallow water? One might hear that fact, and conclude that deeper water is safer. The reality is that sharks attack swimmers where the swimmers are, and most swimmers are in shallow water. The water depth is inconsequential; other factors such as feeding cycles, time of the day, bright colors or blood in the water are causative.

Another error comes in drawing conclusions from "anecdotal incidences". Anecdotal means a single observation or event. One experience does not equal a truth. "Grandma ate garlic for a week and her aches went away." While this may be true, there is no cause and effect relationship. In your healthcare, following this type of logic can result in quackery, delayed treatment or worse. In medicine, for a study to be valid, it must be well designed, large in scope, decisive, repeatable in results and critically reviewed by experts in that specialty, known as peers. This peer review is why using qualified resources like www.webMD.com or www.nih.gov is absolutely essential.

Steps in the Scientific Method

The specifics will vary depending on the nature of the study, but the basics are:

• Observation and gathering relevant data.

• Formulation of hypothesis (theory explaining cause and effect).

• Design experiment which must isolate the one crucial variable you are examining. There can be no other variables. There can be no bias by subjects or by examiner.

• Run experiment. Must be valid and repeatable.

• Analyze data: Results must be statistically significant, i.e. not attributable purely to chance.

• Conclusion: Your hypothesis has been proven or disproved.

• Peer Review.

Applications of the Scientific Method

The scientific method has relevance far beyond the hard sciences. Even if you don't pursue a career in the sciences, understanding the scientific method will make you a better thinker, voter, citizen and consumer. In every phase of life, people will try to persuade you to their point of view. Politicians, lobbyists, financial advisors and salespeople will present their ideas, supported by facts and figures. It is incumbent upon you to be able to rationally sort through the lies to find the truth. This is especially true in evaluating healthcare related issues in the lay press, advertising and other information sources. There is a vast amount of misinformation presented to the public; some is well intentioned and some is pure quackery. Only the scientific method can sift the wheat from the chaff.

A Guiding Principle:

When evaluating new ideas or opinions, consider the credentials of the source.

Finally, an important corollary principle of the scientific method: Scrutinize both the education and the experience of the "expert". Have they trained at a reputable, respected institution and received legitimate credentials in their field? And then, after training, have they actually had significant personal experience in the field? Often they will not fulfill these criteria, and often they will have ulterior motives. This is especially critical in the digital age when the internet permits any member of the public to expound on matters in which they have absolutely no expertise. We are doctors, and if we were to begin advising you on how to fly aircraft, you would be wise to stay on the ground. And you would also be wise to take healthcare advice from doctors and healthcare professionals, not from pharmaceutical companies, misguided celebrities, internet blogs, friends or random strangers.

Reliable Internet Health Resources

During the process of researching and writing this book the authors and contributors used medical textbooks, journals and internet resources. We found, not surprisingly, that the internet has a vast amount of dangerous misinformation presented as medical fact. And even the national media will give exposure, and thereby credence, to unsupported or undocumented medical news. Your health is precious, and following unsound medical advice can have tragic consequences. Therefore, it is essential that you only use reliable and responsible, physician peer reviewed medical information in making your healthcare decisions. Your first resource will always be your personal physician. However, ultimately your health is your responsibility and the more you know the better choices you will make.

US Government Websites

www.nih.gov National Institutes of Health. Health A–Z.

www.cdc.gov Centers for Disease Control.

www.nlm.nih.gov National Library of Medicine.

www.healthfinder.gov General health information.

Health Information Websites

www.webMD.com The leading healthcare portal.

www.medscape.com WebMD's site for healthcare professionals.

www.eMedicine.com Detailed clinical information for healthcare professionals.

www.mayoclinic.com Clinical experts from the Mayo Clinic.

www.merckmanuals.com The world's best selling medical textbook.

www.americanheart.org Dedicated to cardiovascular health.

www.diabetes.org American Diabetes Association.

HEALTH

"The greatest wealth is health."

Virgil   70 BC-19 BC

Medical History and Physician Exam

When you are sick and seek the care of a medical doctor, you enter the healthcare system. Although healthcare in America is unquestionably the best in the world, it isn't perfect. Doctors and nurses are charged with seeing more patients in a shorter time frame than ever before. You need to be your own advocate, armed with a sound understanding of your own medical status and knowledge of how the healthcare system works. In order to do this, you must first understand how physicians diagnose and treat disease so you can give them the information necessary to help you.

SOAP – Physicians use the SOAP approach to evaluate patients. It is comprised of recording the patient's *Subjective* feelings (history of illness, symptoms), *Objective* findings (clinical signs, laboratory data, x-ray findings), reaching an *Assessment* or diagnosis and finally selecting a treatment *Plan*. In this process, the patient's input is a critical major determinant in the final diagnosis and treatment.

Medical History and Vital Signs

A clear, concise and ordered narrative of your subjective findings is absolutely essential in communicating with your primary care physician (PCP), and even more important in the ER when communicating with caregivers unfamiliar with you. A jumbled, incomplete and inaccurate medical history is an obstacle to providing you with correct treatment. The better you are at communicating history, symptoms and signs to your healthcare provider, the better they will be able to help you.

Basic Medical History

Your basic medical history should begin with your date of birth, blood type, allergies and medications and significant medical/surgical history. You should also have your PCP's name and telephone number, so that they can be reached in an emergency. Your medication list is more important than you think. Every medicine, pill, supplement, vitamin or herbal remedy should be listed. Even innocuous vitamins will interact with, amplify or block the effect of pharmaceuticals or anesthetics that your physician may need to utilize. Not knowing this information is forcing your doctor to fly blind, and the results can be hazardous to your health. Your treatment is going to be only as good as the information you provide. This basic medical history is the <u>absolute minimum,</u> and should be carried on a laminated card in your wallet, purse or on your phone. Additionally, keep an updated, full medical history handy, especially if you have any significant medical condition. An example of the Basic Medical History is shown below. Go to <u>www.ydkWydk.com</u> for the Full Medical History Form.

• Keep a personal medical file with copies of laboratory reports, radiology reports, diagnoses, medications and surgical history.

BASIC MEDICAL HISTORY

John Doe   PCP: Jane Smith, MD
                                (409) 555-1212

DOB: Jan 1, 1991   Blood Type: B+

Allergies: Penicillin

Medical Conditions: Asthma

Surgeries: Appendectomy 8/2005
                                St. Mary's Hospital

Medications: Albuterol as needed

                                Multivitamin daily

Alcohol, Tobacco, Drug Use: None

Choosing a Primary Care Physician (PCP)

- Choose a PCP <u>now</u>, not when you are sick and forced to decide recklessly. Any time you move, find a new PCP and transfer your medical records as soon as possible. Establishing continuity of care is critical to the quality of treatment you receive from the system.

- Read and understand your health insurance coverage or other ways to pay for healthcare (student health services). You can discuss details with your health plan or someone in your doctor's office.

- Check with your insurance plan for a list of PCP gatekeepers.

- Call a physician specialist's office, such as a cardiologist, and ask for an unbiased referral to a PCP. Ask them who their doctor is. Check local magazines/papers for "Best Doctors List".

- Ask your friends and family for recommendations.

- Check on the internet to be sure your doctor is board certified. Board eligible means that they are eligible to take the board certification examination but have not taken the test. If they are board certified, they have taken and passed the examination.

- Go online to your state licensing site and check your doctor's credentials and any history of complaints or disciplinary actions.

- Go online to the National Data Bank <u>www.npdb-hipdb.hrsa.gov/</u>.

- Go to the doctor's website.

- If the physician or the office doesn't meet your expectations, find one who will.

What to Do When You Get Sick

- Always know your PCP's office phone number. Call their office for advice, referrals and questions.

- Go to the college health clinic for care. Your school will have a nurse and perhaps a doctor on staff.

- An urgent care clinic associated with the local hospital for medical care is a good option. These facilities are managed and regulated by the local hospital and therefore have an easy referral system to other hospital facilities (x-ray, labs, specialists, surgery).

- If you cannot obtain care in a clinic setting, go to the local emergency room.

- If you feel you have a life threatening medical emergency, call 911 or go to the local hospital emergency room immediately.

Making a Doctor's Appointment

- If you are sick and simple measures do not improve your condition, go immediately to your campus health clinic, an ambulatory care clinic (Doc in the box) or your PCP.

- For routine visits, make 8AM appointment if possible. The first appointment of the day is usually on time, the office is the cleanest, the staff is fresh and no one is rushed with the schedule.

- If you are making an appointment for an afternoon consultation, ask for the first appointment time in the afternoon. Once again, you will be seen first and no one is rushing.

- Never use your Social Security number; your insurance can be processed without this information.

- When you visit for the appointment, look at the office for cleanliness, up to date equipment, cheerful and competent staff. If you do not feel comfortable, find another doctor.

Your Doctor's Appointment

Prepare for your doctor's visit well and optimize the time you have. Excellent communication means a better understanding of your condition, and better treatment. Maximize the interaction.

- Bring your Full Medical History Form, <u>updated and accurate</u>.

- Bring a trusted family member or friend with you to the appointment.

- Prepare for your appointment. Know your medical history, insurance coverage, current medications, allergies and details of the reason for your visit. Write down any questions you may have for the doctor in advance.

- Be on time for your appointment and be prepared to wait; your doctor has other patients who often put him behind schedule.

- See a PCP for your basic care and as an entry into the referral system. Ask your doctor for a referral to a specialist for any surgical treatment or complicated illness.

- Keep your questions and answers short and to the point. Focus on the problem.

- Ask if there are any alternative treatments.

- Ask the doctor "What would you do if I was your daughter/son?"

- Ask the doctor "How many of these procedures have you done?"

- If treatment is not an emergency, consider a second opinion.

Your Physician's Examination

Physicians use a standardized approach to analyze an illness and arrive at a diagnosis and treatment. The following data will be recorded in detail:

Current Complaint: Your medical problem (i.e. nosebleed).

History of the Present Illness: This is an accurate account of the current complaint. The format of: What, Where, When, Why and How is a good start. Have you ever had nose bleeds before? What caused the nose to bleed? Trauma or spontaneous? Where is the blood coming from? Right or left nostril? When did the bleeding start? One hour or ten hours ago? Did it slow down, stop, restart? Was the bleeding consistent? How much blood was on the tissue? What did you do to try to stop it? What makes it better? Or worse? Often it helps in ER situations to have family or friends compile this for the RN or MD. If it is a routine office visit, write it out in advance and be as thorough as possible.

Symptoms: Symptoms are subjective (what you feel). Nausea, dizziness, chills, sore throat, pain, blurry vision or headache are examples. By describing these sensations to your physician, you help shed light on the problem.

Signs: Signs are objective findings (what you see). Bleeding, diarrhea, pale skin tone, vomiting, loss of consciousness are examples. This is the second step in diagnosis, and accuracy is key.

Medical and Surgical History: This is your prepared and documented medical history, and can be printed or in digital format. It may be simple such as a history of asthma and removal of wisdom teeth or complex with multiple illnesses and surgeries. Again, what may seem insignificant to you could be of critical importance, so be thorough.

Family Medical History: A review of any significant illnesses of your family to determine if there are any hereditary diseases or predispositions to consider during your treatment.

Review of Systems: In this phase, the RN or MD will discuss every major body function in appropriate detail to determine if there are clues or existing or past problems that relate to your current complaint, or affect your hospitalization or treatment in some way. Again, information is power. The more the medical team knows about your total health, the better they can treat you.

Up to this point, the responsibility is yours to provide accurate and reliable data from which the healthcare personnel will act. The next step will be a physical examination in appropriate depth and detail and lab or radiological examination. Very often, a physician armed with an excellent history from you will be able to reach a diagnosis without the need of unnecessary, costly or invasive tests. Physicians have a tremendous advantage over veterinarians….we can talk intelligently with our patients.

Physical Examination: Your physician will perform a limited or full physical examination to obtain more objective findings (such as wheezing or heart murmur). In addition, he may order laboratory tests (blood, urine, sputum) or radiographic examination (X-ray, CT, MRI). Always ask if these tests are necessary and if there is an alternative. Always shield your reproductive organs from radiation with a lead apron.

Assessment and Plan: From the above information, the physician uses a decision algorithm to determine his assessment or diagnosis, which may include several possible diseases (such as strep throat, mono or viral pharyngitis for a sore throat) that will be narrowed down with further laboratory tests. Once the assessment has been made, your physician will present the treatment plan with prescriptions, recommendations, additional tests or a referral to a specialist. This is the time to ask questions about the diagnosis, alternative treatment and referrals to specialists.

Vital Signs

Your vital signs are the clues to what is going on in your body, and how your body is coping with the stress of your current illness. A record of vital signs is helpful information to give to the doctor, and your vital signs will be monitored during your visit or hospital stay. Astute clinicians can tell an astonishing amount simply from observing your vital signs.

Vital Signs: Temperature, Blood Pressure, Pulse, Respiratory Rate

Temperature – Take with a digital thermometer and record the T° (in Fahrenheit or Centigrade) and time. Keep a record of all temperatures taken during your illness. Normal is 98.6° F or 37°C.

Medical Alert: Temperatures and Fevers

Do not fixate on the level of T°. An elevated temperature is the body's normal response to stress and an infection. As your T° rises, your immune system becomes activated and more effective in eliminating the invading pathogens. At higher T°, the body's white blood cells and enzymes are more efficient in killing viruses and bacteria. However, there is a point when elevated T° becomes dangerous and must be treated. Consult your physician.

Blood Pressure – A digital automatic BP cuff is adequate for home use. Normal is a systolic pressure of less than 120mmHg and a diastolic pressure of less than 80mmHg.

Pulse – Learn to take your pulse at your wrist (radial artery). Do not take your pulse at your neck. Count for a full minute. Normal rate is between 50-100 beat per minute. Well conditioned athletes may have an even lower heart rate.

Respiratory Rate – Simply count the number of breaths per minute. Normal rate is 8-12 breaths per minute.

First Aid

First aid can be defined as assistance provided by a layperson for treatment or stabilization. It originates with medieval knights such as the Knights Hospitaller, and evolved into the Red Cross and other worldwide organizations whose protocols are shown here.

Protocols

It should be noted that there are three protocols in CPR and First Aid: Untrained Layman, Trained Layman, and Healthcare Professional.

Due to complexity we present only the basics for the untrained layman, and recommend further complete training.

An accredited course in CPR, AED and First Aid is invaluable.

www.heart.org

www.redcross.org

Principles of First Aid

- Save lives of the victim, the responder, and bystanders. Use caution.

- Prevent further harm: Stabilize victim, alert medical professionals.

- Promote recovery: Dress wounds, stop bleeding, render aid.

First and foremost: Assess the situation. Stay calm. Go slow. Tragically, first responders have been killed or injured in roadside accidents or volatile domestic situations. Be careful.

Universal Precautions

The practice of "Universal Precautions" was implemented in healthcare as a method to reduce risk of blood borne and airborne infections (HIV/AIDS, hepatitis, TB). Patients may not reveal or even know they are infected. By assuming that every patient could be infected and using precautions in all patients, risk is greatly lowered. The portal of entry of disease can be the mouth, nose, eyes, mucosa or small, even microscopic cuts in the skin or mucosa. The goal is to protect these areas from contact or splash exposure. The other concern is sharps: any needle, knife, razor or pin that can penetrate skin and carry disease to the bloodstream.

HIV/AIDS, hepatitis and other diseases are transmitted by blood and bodily fluids: semen, vaginal secretions, breast milk, saliva, tears. By wearing barrier fabrics, gloves, masks and eye protection, healthcare personnel minimize risk. While this is unrealistic for laypeople, it is wise to use caution if you render first aid, especially to strangers. Further, the increasing incidence of tuberculosis in the indigent, homeless[1] and immigrants[2] calls for greater caution in urban settings.

General Precautions

Biohazards

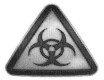

Blood, Bandages, Band-Aids, Tampons, Tissues, Etc.

• Keep gloves, mask and glasses in car/home first aid kit.

• Never allow exposure to blood, body fluids.

• Handle biohazards properly: Use gloves, dispose in plastic bag.

• Immediately wash hands or shower.

• Wash clothing after exposure.

---

1   CDC MMWR/41(RR-5);001

2   www.lungusa.org

Cardiopulmonary Resuscitation (CPR)

Adult Cardiopulmonary Resuscitation CPR

Cardiac arrest is the most common cause of death in the United States. CPR is a life saving technique that combines chest compressions and mouth to mouth resuscitation (M2M or rescue breathing) to maintain blood flow during cardiac events. In October 2010, the protocols for Basic CPR were simplified and M2M was abandoned.[3] Survival rates without M2M are comparable, and speed and efficiency is improved. The old, familiar ABC (Airway Breathing Circulation) sequence was updated to:

CAB : Circulation – Airway – Breathing

This is a summary of the steps for providing Adult CPR by the untrained; however there is no substitute for taking the American Heart Association course and keeping up to date. Get trained at www.heart.org.

Hands Only Basic Resuscitation for Untrained Laypersons

• Assess the victim for response.

• If no response, shout for help.

• Call 911 and get an automated external defibrillator if nearby.

• Immediately begin chest compressions. Kneel by side, heel of palm on sternum two fingers above inferior tip, fingers interlocked. With arms straight, elbows locked, use body weight to compress at least 2" and at a rate of at least 100 compressions per minute. Push hard and fast, allowing the chest to recoil after compression.

• When AED arrives, use as directed (see Automated External Defibrillator).

• Continue until advanced life support providers arrive.

An Outstanding Resource

http://handsonlycpr.org

Videos, online instruction and free smartphone and iphone apps for CPR.

---

3   M2M is retained in the protocols for Trained Laypersons and Healthcare Providers.

Automated External Defibrillator (AED)

The AED is a technological jewel, a battery powered computer that diagnoses arrhythmias and will shock the heart if, and only if, necessary. It is incredibly simple. When opened, the AED will prompt you through setup and use. Lives have been saved by untrained responders who have never used AEDs before. However, we strongly recommend that you complete an American Heart Association sponsored CPR/AED course. www.heart.org.

Time is Life

Ventricular arrhythmias result in brain death in minutes.
Prompt use of the AED is critical.

CPR must be initiated before using the AED

AED Overview

COMPRESSIONS MUST CONTINUE WHILE PREPARING AED

- Locate AED ASAP; survival rate is higher with early intervention.
- Turn on AED.
- Most AEDs will "talk" and give you instructions.
- Remove patient's shirt, underwire bra, piercings, and jewelry.
- Wipe patients chest dry (no moisture).
- Apply pads to bare chest (see diagram in AED).
- Pad 1 – on upper right chest.
- Pad 2 – on lower left side of chest.
- Plug pad connectors into AED.
- Let AED analyze heart rhythm.
- Stand clear, do not touch patient.
- Deliver shock as prompted by AED.
- If no shock indicated, continue CPR.

   Prompt, skilled CPR and defibrillation greatly improves survival rate and recovery.

Heimlich Maneuver or Abdominal Thrusts

The Universal Choking Sign: Victim clutches his throat with both hands.

Abdominal thrusts, or the Heimlich Maneuver, is a technique for clearing an obstructed airway (choking) in a conscious victim which if left untreated may result in death. In adults, this occurs most often while eating. The exact technique is taught at a First Aid/ CPR course by the American Red Cross. This training is priceless; even 10 year old children have been able to save lives using the techniques taught by the Red Cross.

Overview of Technique

Not intended as a substitute for Red Cross training. Go to www.redcross.org.

- Stand behind the individual who is choking and inform them what you are doing. Get their consent to proceed. Have a bystander call 911.

- Deliver 5 back blows with the heel of your hand between the victim's shoulder blades.

- Deliver 5 abdominal thrusts (the Heimlich Maneuver) to the victim.

  1. Tip the victim forward slightly at the waist.

  2. Place your arms around the victim's waist below the rib cage.

  3. Make a fist in the center with your thumb towards the victim; place your other hand over your fist tightly.

  4. Deliver upward and inward thrusts to the abdomen, as if trying to lift the victim off the ground. This will push the diaphragm upward, increasing pressure in the lungs and simulate a forceful cough to expel the airway obstruction.

- Repeat the cycle of 5 back blows followed by 5 abdominal thrusts as necessary until obstruction is dislodged or patient becomes unconscious.

- If patient becomes unconscious, lay gently on the floor and carefully check mouth. Remove obstruction if possible, begin CPR. Chest compressions may dislodge the foreign object; check the mouth frequently.

Self Administered Heimlich

If you are alone and choking, the back blows are impossible to do; go straight to the Heimlich Maneuver. This can be done solo with the help of a countertop, table or chair.

- Place a fist with your thumb directed inward, just above your navel.

- Place your other hand over the fist and deliver upward and inward thrusts to abdomen. If unable to dislodge object, use countertop, table or chair.

• Bend over or drive your body onto a table, countertop or chair to force your fist up and inward.

This technique is worth learning and practicing. Choking on food, vitamin pills, medications and other foreign bodies can occur even in healthy adults. Being prepared could save your life.

Bleeding

When you are living and experiencing life, the occasional injury will occur. Minor abrasions and lacerations can be treated with simple first aid techniques. Serious injuries should be stabilized for transport to the ER. The best strategy is prevention (Kevlar® glove) and caution when handling sharp things.

Basic Principles

Bleeding should be controlled as rapidly as possible. Blood vessels are self-sealing, but clotting takes time. Do not panic. Excitement raises blood pressure and renews bleeding. The best technique is gentle pressure, just enough to stop the bleeding, directly on the bleeding area for 10 minutes, by the clock. Repeatedly inspecting the wound removes the clot and restarts bleeding.

• Apply gentle pressure directly on the point of bleeding for 10 minutes.

• Elevate the wound above the level of the heart.

• Calm and reassure the victim. Give it time.

Arterial Bleeding

Arterial bleeding will be bright red, brisk and pulsatile. This is serious and requires immediate medical treatment. Call 911. Apply direct pressure, just enough to stop the bleeding, directly on the bleeding area for 10 minutes, by the clock. If bleeding has stopped, bandage and transport.

Medical Alert: Tourniquet Use

USE ONLY IN LIFE THREATENING SITUATIONS

In limb injuries (never use on neck), a tourniquet may be needed in life threatening bleeding if direct pressure fails and as the last resort. If possible, call 911 for medical advice before use. The wider and thicker the tourniquet is, the better. Tourniquets must be used with great care. If improperly applied they can cut off all blood supply to the limb and cause nerve, muscle and tissue damage, amputation or death. Tighten the tourniquet just enough to stop the bleeding. Record the time the tourniquet was applied *and immediately call 911* for further medical treatment.

Minor Wounds

Bleeding from veins and capillaries will be slow, red/dark red and non-pulsatile. Gently cleanse the wound with clean tap or bottled water and mild soap or antiseptic wash.

Medical Alert: Povidone Iodine (Betadine®)

This thick brown liquid is an excellent surgical prep solution, but should be used only on intact skin. If used on open wounds or mucosa, it may kill tissue, increase infection rate and delay healing. J&J Antiseptic Wash or copious clear water is better for cleansing open wounds.

Avoid using harsh antiseptics (hydrogen peroxide, alcohol, povidone iodine) on open wounds as they kill tissue as well as microbes[4]. An abundance of fresh clean water and gentle cleansing will remove dirt, gravel, debris and contamination. It is important to get all foreign material out of the wound, as it may cause infection, scarring or tattooing as the wound heals. Use gentle direct pressure to stop bleeding. Apply a light coat of bacitracin and cover with a non-adherent dressing. Bandages should give gentle pressure to the wound to protect the dressing and minimize bleeding. Consult your physician for further care specific to your injury.

Wound Care

The goal is to promote healing, reduce pain, control infection and absorb fluid. Change dressing frequently, observe the wound and reapply bacitracin. Dispose of all bandages in a sanitary fashion.

Ice Packs

Ice packs can reduce swelling, inflammation and pain in many injuries, especially in the first 72 hours. Keys to maximize results:

• Never fall asleep with ice pack on skin.

• Always place washcloth between ice pack and skin.

• Use ice pack for 15 minutes maximum.

• Frozen peas in zip seal bag are excellent, reusable and lightweight. Perfect for face.

---

4 Kramer SA. "Effect of Povidone-iodine on wound healing: a review." J Vasc Nurs. 1999 Mar;17(1):17-23

The "Tourniquet Effect" of Dressings

When bandaging an extremity/limb/finger/appendage, avoid circumferential wrapping, especially with tape and compressive elastic wraps. Swelling causes a circumferential dressing to become a tourniquet, often unobserved, and can result in tissue death, gangrene or amputation. Apply dressings to limbs loosely, and monitor constantly.

Most wounds will heal uneventfully, but be vigilant for the warning signs:

• Fever

• Redness or pain that is increasing or spreading.

• Increasing or changing discharge: yellow/green/foul smelling.

If any of these signs appear, seek medical attention immediately.

Basic Infectious Disease

The main groups of infectious disease causing entities, listed in increasing order of size and cellular complexity, are: prions, viruses, bacteria, fungi and parasites. Prions are protein molecules that cause extremely rare degenerative brain diseases. Fungi, which include yeasts and molds, are common but rarely life threatening. Parasites can be single celled organisms like protozoa all the way up to complex organisms like tapeworms. Fortunately parasites are relatively rare in the US. The vast majority of serious infectious disease is caused by viruses or bacteria, and in some illnesses it is difficult to tell if the cause is viral or bacterial. This is critical because although the symptoms are the same, the treatment is different.

Viruses

Viruses are microscopic infectious agents consisting only of their genetic code and a capsule. They cannot reproduce on their own and require a living cell in which to replicate. They are very simple, very hardy, and very efficient. Typically, a virus will attach to a living cell, inject its genes and proteins into the cell, and take over the cell's function. It will then multiply until the cell bursts with viral offspring. Viruses cause tremendous human misery because antibiotics do not kill them. Vaccines and antiviral drugs offer some protection; however, viruses are constantly adapting and developing resistant strains. Prevention by hygiene and sanitary practices is the key. Viral Diseases: Smallpox, Bird Flu, Swine Flu, Common Cold, Influenza, Hepatitis, AIDS.

Bacteria

Bacteria are simple, single celled organisms that can reproduce. They are ubiquitous; on our skin, within our bodies, in our food. The vast majority are harmless, and many are actually beneficial and essential to health. However, when the normal bacterial flora of our bodies is overrun by virulent bacteria, disease occurs. Bacterial Diseases: Cholera, Dysentery, Plague, TB, Toxic Shock Syndrome, Strep Throat, Methicillin Resistant Staph Aureus (MRSA).

Medical Alert: Improper Use of Antibiotics

A very real cause of the increasing threat of aggressive killer bacteria like MRSA is the improper use of antibiotics coupled with increasing use of antibacterial soaps. Both these trends act to selectively breed more resistant bacteria and exacerbate viral disease. The use of antibiotics in viral infections or the use of the incorrect antibiotic in a bacterial infection only worsens the condition of the patient and breeds a more dangerous and resistant germ. Never self medicate or use leftover antibiotics to blindly treat an infection. Consult your physician.

Contagious Disease

Bacteria, fungi and viruses often spread easily from person to person in close quarters (dorm rooms, airplanes, bathrooms, restaurants, apartments). Good habits can help you avoid illness.

Vectors of Disease Transmission

Airborne – cough/sneeze/speech via infectious droplets.

Direct Contact – touching infected person or surface.

Fecal-Oral – poor hygiene, sexual contact or food preparation.

Blood borne – contact with blood or body fluids.

Prevention

- Avoid touching your face, mouth, nose or eyes with your hands. This is the most common portal of entry for contagious disease.

- Wash your hands before meals and any time you have contacted someone who is sick or has flu symptoms.

- Never use handkerchiefs; carrying excreta in your pocket is unhealthy. Use disposable tissues and discard immediately after use, then wash your hands.

- Avoid contact with the public bathroom fixtures (door knobs, faucets, toilet handle), as most people do not wash their hands.

- Use seat covers in public toilets, try not to make any skin to toilet contact.

- Use alcohol based hand sanitizers when unable to wash hands, when bathrooms are unclean or when on an airplane.

- Do not share food or drink. Politely decline when offered to "try" someone's meal or beverage, you are also trying their saliva. Avoid buffet meals or be in line first.

- Never eat from communal bowls like bar peanuts, pretzels, etc. Hand-mouth-hand from many patrons contaminates these bowls with saliva.

- Eat at clean well known restaurants (more food turnover, less spoilage). Open kitchens are best; you can see them cook and they are forced to keep a clean environment.

- Do not share your toothbrush or store your toothbrush in the same cup as your roommate; either habit will inoculate you with his/her bacteria/fungus/virus from their saliva.

- Clean your dishes, glasses and coffee mugs with soap and hot water.

- Wear sandals or slippers when in public bathrooms and showers (dorm, pool, beach, locker room). Athlete's foot fungus (*tinea*) thrives in these environments.

- Do not share razor blades or electric razors. You are mixing blood and putting yourself at risk for hepatitis, HIV and other blood borne diseases.

- Practice abstinence or safe sex. Use a latex condom every time you engage in oral, vaginal or anal sex. STDs occur from all types of sexual contact.

- Do not share makeup, lipstick, lip balm, eye shadow or deodorant. Don't borrow or let others borrow your personal items.

- If you have a cut or abrasion, immediately clean with soap and water and disinfect with antibacterial cleanser. Use liquid wound sealants.

- Never wear underwear or socks two days in a row.

- Wash your bedding and towels in hot 130°F water and bleach once a week.

- Wash your pillow once a month.

- Shower and shampoo after working out and/or at the end of a day out in public. Use unscented soap and warm water, clean thoroughly.

Methicillin Resistant Staphylococcus Aureus (MRSA)

Staphylococcus Aureus is part of the normal bacterial flora of the human body, and usually is harmless. However, due to decades of widespread use of antibiotics and the extremely short life cycle and rapid evolution of bacteria, drug resistant strains of staph have developed. MRSA is a particularly virulent and communicable pathogen, and it is estimated that 1% of the population are carriers. MRSA began in the hospital setting, where use of antibiotics and antiseptics as well as patient turnover bred the germ, named Hospital Acquired MRSA. Recently, a disturbing increase in the Community Acquired MRSA (CA-MRSA) form has been seen.

CA-MRSA

This strain is of great concern to everyone, and especially to college students, military personnel, athletes and anyone living in crowded conditions such as dorms or fraternities and sororities. CA-MRSA primarily affects patients in their twenties.

Causes and Risk Factors

- Athletics and contact sports
- Gyms and workout facilities
- Communal living, daycare facilities
- Military personnel
- Tattoos
- Sharing personal items: razors, towels, equipment, gear, clothing

Symptoms and Signs

- First sign is a skin infection.
- Fever, chills, headache, rash, joint pain may occur.
- Skin infection worsens and spreads. Abscesses form.
- Blood borne spread of disease to heart, kidney, lungs, joints.

Treatment

Diagnosis will be done by exam and culture. Treatment may require antibiotics or hospitalization. The full course of antibiotics must be taken, if prescribed. Often a patient will feel better after a few days, and cease taking the antibiotic; this only allows more aggressive and resistant bacteria to survive, a potentially lethal development.

Prevention

Prevention is absolutely essential, as MRSA may eventually become untreatable.

• Always wash hands, especially after hospital, gym, exposure to crowds.

• Wear gym gloves and clean off gym equipment before and after use.

• Shower after workouts, athletics, and exposure to crowds or travel.

• Never share personal items: razors, towels, athletic gear, etc.

• Avoid community or unclean whirlpools, spas, saunas, tubs.

• Wound care: Keep wounds covered, frequently change bandages, dispose of them in a sanitary fashion, and never touch others' soiled bandages.

• Launder clothes, towels, bedding frequently and properly.

Hand Washing

Frequent, thorough hand washing is the best way to avoid common communicable diseases, yet hand washing is often done incorrectly. Adults touch their hands to their faces an average of 30 times hourly, a primary vector of disease transmission. While it is unnecessary to do a full surgical scrub, proper technique makes a difference.

Surgical Dictum: *Dilution is the Solution to Pollution*

Bacteria are ubiquitous and usually harmless, but potentially lethal pathogens like *E.coli* and *Salmonella* are everywhere as well. The goal is to limit the exposure to the pathogen by keeping clean.

Always wash before: eating or preparing food, contact with a sick or infected person, cleaning or dressing a wound, brushing your teeth or putting in contact lenses.

Always wash after: touching bare skin, shaking hands, handling food or raw meat/poultry (salmonella), using the toilet/changing diapers, coughing, sneezing or using a tissue, touching a sick, injured or infected person, touching shoes, rags or garden tools, touching animals or animal items. Be especially careful when traveling; airplanes, airports, hotels and bathrooms can be contaminated.

Technique

Warm water and regular soap is best. Antibacterial soaps are useful for special situations, but may actually increase our susceptibility to pathogens if used regularly.

- Wash with warm water for 20 seconds (sing *"Happy Birthday"* twice).

- Clean wrists, hands, webs, palms and especially nails.

- Rinse thoroughly. Grab towel without touching dispenser.

- When in a public restroom, dry hands with towel and use towel on handle to open door.

- When traveling, take clean handkerchief for facilities with no towel or air dryers.

If soap and water aren't available, use a hand sanitizer. Be sure the alcohol level is 60% or more. Thoroughly wet hands with the gel, then rub over entire hands until dry. Do not overuse these products, as they can cause drying and cracking of skin which creates a portal for infection.

Allergies

An allergy occurs when a foreign substance or allergen reacts with your immune system. The immune system normally protects our bodies from invading bacteria or viruses but some individuals react to otherwise harmless allergens in an exaggerated fashion called an "allergic reaction". The allergen can be a food, medication, pet dander, insect bite, pollen, cosmetics, metal or other substances. Most allergies are mild in nature and may resolve or diminish with time; however a severe, life threatening allergic reaction called anaphylaxis can occur resulting in low blood pressure, airway constriction, loss of consciousness and death. Most anaphylactic reactions are caused by food allergies and insect bites.

Common Causes of Allergic Reactions

- Food allergies – eggs, peanuts, shellfish, soy.
- Insect sting – bee, wasp.
- Hay fever or allergic rhinitis – pollen, grass.
- Drug allergy – penicillin, sulfa drugs, iodine.
- Other causes – latex, pet dander, dust mites, mold.

Symptoms of a Mild Allergy

- Itchy or watery eyes
- Itching of nose, mouth, throat or skin
- Red and swollen eyes (conjunctivitis)
- Runny nose
- Skin rash
- Hives or welts
- Headache
- Diarrhea or vomiting
- Coughing or wheezing
- Atopic dermatitis (eczema)

Treatment of Mild Allergic Reaction

Avoid allergens and seek medical evaluation for a complete exam, allergy testing, blood test and the most effective medication for your allergies:

- Antihistamines (Benadryl, Zyrtec, Claritin). Available over the counter and by prescription. These medications block histamine release and lessen symptoms.

- Corticosteriods (hydrocortisone, prednisone, Advair). Available over the counter and by prescription. These are potent anti-inflammatory medications but have side effects. Use with caution and physician supervision.

- Leukotriene inhibitors (Singulair, Accolate). Available by prescription only. Leukotrienes are synthesized in the antigen-antibody interaction and cause airway constriction. Inhibiting leukotrienes opens airways.

- Immunotherapy (allergy shots). Given at a physician's office. A gradual introduction of the allergen to your immune system diminishes the allergic response.

Symptoms of a Severe Allergy

- Difficulty breathing

- Swelling of mouth, tongue or throat, blocking normal breathing

- Rapid and weak heart beat

- Lightheadedness or loss of consciousness due to low blood pressure

- Hives, flushing of the skin or pale skin

- Nausea, vomiting or diarrhea

- Shock

Treatment of a Severe Allergic Reaction

- Call 911 and seek immediate medical attention. Do not try to wait and see if goes away. Call for ambulance or go to the ER.

- While you are waiting for the ambulance, take 25mg to 50mg of the antihistamine Benadryl.

- If you have wheezing, use an inhaler (albuterol) if available.

- If you have been prescribed an epinephrine kit (Epi-Pen), use as directed. This kit is used only in life threatening allergic reactions. Effective and fast acting, causing increase of blood pressure, opening of airway and lung passages. Given in ER by physician or self administered as an injection to outer thigh with Epi-Pen device.

- If symptoms resolve with Epi-Pen, you should still seek immediate medical care as symptoms may return.

Asthma

Asthma is a chronic inflammatory disease causing swelling and narrowing of the airway (bronchospasm) with wheezing, coughing and difficulty breathing. Asthma affects 34 million people nationally with a high incidence among elite athletes. It is one of the most common causes of emergency room visits and there are approximately 5000 asthma related deaths per year.

Causes and Triggers

- Cold, dry air
- High pollen counts, animal dander
- Air pollution, smog, dust, smoke
- Emotional stress, physical exercise
- Food additives (sulfites), aspirin or NSAIDs
- Concurrent respiratory infection, common cold, allergies

Symptoms and Signs

- Wheezing
- Coughing without mucus production
- Chest tightness or pain
- Shortness of breath, rapid pulse, anxiety

Diagnosis

If you develop asthma, seek medical care immediately. Evaluation includes allergy testing, a chest x-ray, pulmonary function tests and blood tests.

Treatment

There are two basic types of asthma medications: maintenance drugs to prevent attacks and rescue drugs for acute asthma attacks. Common maintenance medications are inhaled corticosteroids (Flovent, Advair, Pulmicort). These medications reduce inflammation and swelling. The rescue drugs are short acting bronchodilators (Proventil, Ventolin) that relax the airway; they should also be used prior to exercise in patients with exercise induced asthma. Learn how to use the inhaler properly; experts estimate that one in four patients use them incorrectly. Asthma is a chronic disease; adjustment of treatment modalities and regular evaluation by your physician is essential.

Sore Throat

Sore throat (pharyngitis) is a common, usually minor illness that resolves with time. Sore throats are most often a result of either viral or bacterial infections. Viral causes include influenza, "mono" (mononucleosis) and measles. Bacterial causes include strep throat, whooping cough and diphtheria.

Symptoms and Signs

• Pain with swallowing, scratchy throat, swollen neck nodes, enlarged and inflamed tonsils, difficulty eating or speaking are the main symptoms.

• Fever, cough, chills, aches, rash, headache, diarrhea or vomiting may occur.

Causes

Most sore throats are caused by viral infections like the common cold or "mono", a viral illness spread by saliva and called the "kissing disease" for that reason. Mono is usually mild and symptoms last for only 2-4 weeks. Diagnosis is confirmed with blood test (monospot or EBV serology). See Mononucleosis.

Sore throat can also be caused by bacteria, most commonly the streptococcal bacteria. When this occurs, it is called strep throat. It is diagnosed by a "rapid strep test" or a throat culture. Complications of strep throat include sinus infections, tonsillitis, scarlet fever, rheumatic fever and rheumatic heart disease.

Treatment

Most sore throats can be treated at home. Go to your doctor if you have a persistent high fever, are unable to swallow or open your mouth, are not improving after 24 hours, or have difficulty breathing. Treatment will depend upon the cause of your sore throat. Your doctor will examine you and may take blood tests and a throat swab to rule out strep throat. Bacterial infections are treated with antibiotics such as penicillin or azithromycin. Treatment of viral infection is supportive in nature and includes fluids, analgesics/antipyretics (never use aspirin in patients under 20 years old due to Reye's Syndrome), and palliative therapy (throat lozenges). Antibiotics are ineffective against viral infections, and can actually be harmful.

Prevention

Good personal hygiene, proper hand washing and minimizing touching your face, nose, eyes and mouth. See Contagious Disease.

The Common Cold

The common cold is caused by hundreds of different viruses, mainly rhinoviruses and adenoviruses. Because these viruses continually mutate, there is no vaccine or effective medicine for prevention. The illness is confined primarily to the nose and throat. Infection is spread by sneezing, coughing or touching an infected person and then touching your nose, eyes or mouth.

Symptoms

- Sneezing, coughing, runny nose, itchy watery eyes, nasal congestion, sore throat and hoarseness.
- Remember that your cold is most contagious in the first 48 hours of symptoms, so limit your contact with others during that period.

Treatment

- Treatment is symptomatic (aimed at reducing the symptoms).
- Do not use antibiotics unless your doctor has examined you and diagnosed a secondary bacterial infection.
- Use steam vaporizers or saline nasal sprays to open the airway. Use medicated OTC nasal sprays for 3 days only or rebound congestion will occur.
- Rest and get plenty of fluids for hydration. Acetaminophen or ibuprofen for fever and pain relief.
- Consult your physician if you experience: a high, prolonged fever above 102°F or for 3 or more days with fatigue and body aches, symptoms that last for more than 10 days, trouble breathing or shortness of breath, chest pain, confusion, severe or persistent vomiting, swollen glands, fainting, infection spreading to ears, sinuses, lungs. In severe cases, a secondary bacterial infection may occur.

Correct Sneeze/Cough Etiquette

A sneeze or cough sends a huge wet spray of infectious droplets up to 20 feet at a velocity of 100 mph. Cover your mouth and nose with a disposable tissue when you sneeze or cough. Immediately discard the tissue. Wash your hands. If you do not have a tissue, bury your face in the crook of your elbow or your shoulder, and wash up immediately.

Prevention

The only prevention method is good hygiene.

Flu

Influenza or 'flu' is a viral infection of the lungs and airways. There are three types of influenza: A, B, C. Type A causes the most epidemics. Infection begins 24-48 hours after touching an infected person or surface or by inhaling aerosol virus from a cough or sneeze. Secondary bacterial infections can develop and cause more serious problems.

Symptoms

• Fever, chills, shakes, sneezing, sore throat, headache, muscle aches.

• Nasal discharge or productive cough usually not present.

• Dry cough, weakness may occur.

Treatment

• There is no cure for the flu; you treat the symptoms.

• Take your temperature.

• Use acetaminophen (Tylenol®) for fever as directed.

• Take a multivitamin.

• Keep a daily record of the amount of fluid you take in, the medicine you take (so you do not exceed recommended amount) and your temperature.

• Replenish fluids with clear juices, sports drinks or oral hydration fluid.

• Advance your diet from a bland diet (Jell-O, applesauce, broth) to soft diet (soup, eggs, yogurt). Maintain protein and calorie intake.

• Consult your physician if you experience a high, prolonged fever above 102°F or for 3 or more days with fatigue and body aches, symptoms that last for more than 10 days, trouble breathing or shortness of breath, chest pain, fainting, confusion, severe or persistent vomiting, severe sinus pain or swollen glands.

• Antibiotics are not effective but antivirals such as zanamivir may be considered by your doctor.

• Complete recovery usually in 1 to 2 weeks.

Prevention

• Wash your hands often and especially before meals.

• Do not contact your nose, eyes or mouth with your hands.

• Use alcohol hand sanitizers after shaking hands or contact with infected persons.

Consult your physician and consider the annual flu shot.

The best way to avoid the flu is to get the annual influenza vaccine. The vaccine against the latest types of flu becomes available each fall, but you can get it any time throughout the year by injection or nasal spray. Vaccination is convenient, inexpensive and does not require a prescription. Many pharmacies offer walk-in vaccination. The vaccines work by exposing your immune system to an attenuated flu virus and thereby stimulating immunity, much in the same way that actually having a full blown course of the disease does, but without the misery. Vaccine safety and efficiency is carefully monitored by the CDC. www.CDC.gov.

Diagnosis and Treatment:
Common Cold vs. Flu vs. Allergy

Although the common cold and influenza (flu) are both caused by viruses and have similar symptoms, they are completely different diseases. Prevention is difficult. You can get an annual flu shot that protects you from the most prevalent influenza virus but there is no vaccination for the common cold. In the majority of cases, you just treat the symptoms. In severe cases, you should seek medical care.

Both the common cold and the flu can present with: cough, headache, muscle aches, fatigue and stuffy nose/sinus.

Typical Common Cold Symptoms: mainly nose and throat involvement, mild fever (up to 102°F), green or yellow nasal discharge, sore throat, sneezing.

Typical Flu Symptoms: non-productive dry cough, high fever (over 102°F), nausea, chills and sweats, loss of appetite.

Making the diagnosis isn't critical, as the treatment is the same for both:

• Rest. Sleep it off, especially if you have a fever. Rest helps fight infection.

• Take a multivitamin and Vitamin C supplement.

• Drink lots of fluids such as water and clear soups (chicken soup). Fluids keep you hydrated and help your circulatory system fight infection. Hydration also loosens mucus.

• Eat fruits and vegetables high in antioxidants (beta-carotene, Vitamin C, Vitamin E) and bioflavonoids. Antioxidants neutralize free radicals and help you recover from illness faster. Bioflavonoids speed recovery by assisting your immune system. You can find these in citrus, spinach, grapes, cherries, broccoli and other raw fruits and vegetables.

• Take in adequate protein (yogurt, chicken soup, protein shake) to repair cell injury and fight infection.

• Warm black or green tea with honey will relieve your sore throat, loosen mucus and has antioxidants.

• If you are congested, take warm steam shower or use salt water nasal/sinus sprays to loosen secretion.

• Avoid alcohol, tobacco and coffee.

Over The Counter (OTC) Treatment Options

Your cold or flu cannot be cured but you can reduce the symptoms by using OTC medicines. There are many options available in your pharmacy; choose the medicine that treats your symptoms and read the labels carefully. If you have questions, talk to your doctor or pharmacist for advice and recommendations.

Seek professional medical care if you experience:

A high, prolonged fever (above 102°F) for more than three days with fatigue and body aches, symptoms that last for more than 10 days, trouble breathing or shortness of breath, chest pain, fainting, confusion, severe or persistent vomiting, severe sinus pain or swollen glands.

Allergy Versus The Common Cold?

It is often hard to differentiate between an allergy and a cold because the symptoms are very similar. Colds are caused by highly contagious viruses while allergies are caused by normally harmless environmental irritants. Despite the cause, both conditions activate the immune system and release histamine which produces the typical symptoms of sneezing and a runny, stuffy nose. Colds usually occur during the winter while allergies are usually seasonal. However, colds may present with fever, cough, sore throat, general body aches and colored mucus while allergies typically present with itchy, water eyes and clear mucus. These are only guidelines; for further information, consult your physician.

Over the Counter
Analgesics/Antipyretics/NSAIDs

Be aware that high doses of these OTC medications can cause severe organ failure or death. Read the label of every medicine you take. Follow dosage recommendations. Calculate your dosages when using combination medicines. Be extremely careful giving OTC medications to children and consult a pediatrician. Dosage recommendations shown here are for normal healthy adults. For older patients or compromised patients, consult your physician.

Analgesics are medications that relieve pain. Antipyretics are medications that reduce fever. The following medications have both properties.

Acetaminophen

• Acetaminophen (Tylenol). Reduces pain and fever. Effective in 30-60 minutes. Usual dosage is 325-650 mg every 4-6 hours, or 1000 mg 3-4 times daily, not to exceed 3000 mg per day. Works directly in brain to dull pain and reduce fever. Best choice for headaches, but also used for other minor aches and pains. Can cause liver damage if taken excessively or with alcohol.

NSAIDs

The class of non-steroidal anti-inflammatory drugs, NSAIDs, includes many OTC and prescription drugs. All reduce pain, inflammation and fever; however effects vary with each specific drug, and vary from person to person. Inadvertent use of several NSAIDs concurrently can be dangerous. Always take with food, never on an empty stomach.

• Ibuprofen (Advil, Motrin). Reduces pain and fever. Works in 30 minutes. Usual dosage is 200-400 mg every 4 -6 hours, not to exceed 1200 mg per day unless directed by a physician. Works at the site of injury, reducing pain and swelling. Best choice for muscle soreness or injury. May cause stomach upset or ulcers.

• Naproxen (Naprosyn, Aleve). Usual dosage is 200 mg every 8-12 hours with initial dose of 400 mg if desired. Maximum daily dose 600 mg per day unless directed by physician. Often used for arthritis, menstrual cramps and moderate muscle soreness.

• Aspirin (Bayer, Bufferin, Ecotrin). Reduces pain and fever. Strong, long acting (4-7d) anticoagulant. Works in 30-60 minutes. Usual dosage is 325-650 mg every 4-6 hours, not to exceed 4000 mg per day. Will cause stomach upset. Take with 8 oz. water. Never use in children or teenagers due to association with Reye's syndrome.

Combination Medications

Pharmaceutical companies will combine multiple drugs for added effect such as Excedrin Migraine (acetaminophen, aspirin and caffeine) or Tylenol PM (Tylenol and Benadryl). Read the labels and understand what is in the medication and why. For example: Tylenol PM has acetaminophen for minor pain and uses Benadryl's side effect of drowsiness for a sleep aid. Excedrin Migraine combines the synergistic analgesic actions of acetaminophen and aspirin, while caffeine is added for the stimulant effect. These medications should be taken sparingly and with the advice of your physician. Beware that prescription narcotic pain relievers often have OTC analgesic and antipyretic components, and watch total daily dosage of the individual medications carefully.

OTC Cold Medications

Cold medicine is used to relieve the symptoms of the common cold and flu. The four main ingredients in these medications are analgesics/antipyretics, antihistamines, decongestants and cough suppressants/expectorants.

• Analgesics/Antipyretics: acetaminophen (Tylenol), ibuprofen (Advil, Motrin), naprosyn (Aleve) and aspirin (Bayer). These relieve pain and reduce fever. Best choice is an acetaminophen or ibuprofen based combination.

• Antihistamines: dephenhydramine (Benadryl), brompheniramine and chlorpheniramine. These medications block histamine release that is responsible for sneezing and runny nose. Other antihistamines, Claritin and Zyrtec (used for seasonal allergies) are not thought to be effective in the treatment of cold symptoms.

• Decongestants: pseudoephedrine (Sudafed), phenylephrine (Sudafed PE) and oxymetazoline (Afrin). These medications shrink swollen nasal mucosa and improve airflow. Similar to epinephrine, they can cause nervousness, agitation and hypertension. Use with caution and be careful of combination OTC medications. Nasal sprays should not be used for more than 3 days or rebound congestion and physical dependence may occur.

• Antitussives (also called cough suppressants): dextromethorphan which blocks the cough reflex in the brain. Don't take an antitussive if you're coughing up mucus; you want to clear it out.

• Expectorants: guaifenesin acts to help thin mucus so it can be coughed up easily and removed from your airway.

Recommendations: Evaluate your symptoms and take the appropriate combination medication. Carefully monitor your running total dosage of the individual component medications to avoid overdosage.

Herbal and Alternative Medical Remedies

"Alternative Medicine", including naturopathic, homeopathic and herbal supplements and remedies, is a $34B/year industry. While the FDA strictly regulates pharmaceuticals, "natural" remedies are classified as "dietary supplements" and are not well studied, nor do they undergo FDA evaluation for therapeutic efficacy. Long term effects are not well known. Many of these products are manufactured overseas where dosage consistency, quality control and ethical considerations are substandard. Illegal drugs, contaminants, undeclared medications and carcinogens have been found in supplements.

Supplements claim to improve memory and energy, burn fat or improve joint flexibility, even prevent cancer, while the fine print states otherwise. Be wary of supplements claiming to be safe because they are natural or herbal. Hemlock is natural, and poisonous. Pig manure is natural. Natural isn't always safe, or healthy.

A recent study in the British Journal of Clinical Pharmacology[5] looked at ER patients admitted for poisoning and found that over 75% of the weight loss supplements they were taking contained multiple pharmaceutical agents, some of which were illegal, banned or carcinogenic. Sibutramine, fluoxetine (Prozac®), and fenfluramine were all found in supplements, as well as the cancer causing laxative phenolphthalein.

Unfortunately, there are too many contaminated or counterfeit remedies to list here. Go to www.fda.gov for a list of banned and dangerous supplements. The University of Maryland Medical Center www.umm.edu/altmed has an excellent list of herbal alternative medicine supplements and the known risks, side effects and interactions with prescription drugs. Adding remedies with unknown side effects and drug interactions to an existing Rx drug regimen can be dangerous. Your physician and pharmacist cannot predict interactions with unknown or untested substances.

Do not take these supplements if you are: pregnant, breast feeding, hypertensive, having surgery or taking any OTC medications. It is a mistake to underestimate the potential dangers of these substances. There are reported cases of intracranial bleeding in patients taking ginko biloba with ibuprofen. While all medications have risk, untested supplements carry unacceptable risk and should be avoided.

---

5 M. Tang, MD et al. BJCP October 14, 2010 www.bjcp-journal.com

Bird Flu H5N1 and Swine Flu H1N1

Definitions: An epidemic is an increase above normal incidence of a disease; an epidemic that spreads worldwide is a pandemic.

Most experts believe that an influenza pandemic is not only possible, but inevitable and overdue. Since 1900, there have been four influenza pandemics; the most severe was Spanish Flu in 1918 that killed fifty million people. Pandemics occur when a new strain of virus appears to which we have no immunity, usually because the virus spreads to humans from another species. Influenza strains are largely species-specific; they usually only infect one species. However, bird flu and swine flu have both shown the ability to infect humans.

Patient Zero may be someone with a seasonal influenza infection who becomes simultaneously infected with H5N1 and/or H1N1. Within his infected cells, the viruses will exchange genetic material, and the resultant hybrid supervirus will now be able to infect humans. Given that even the relatively mild seasonal flu kills 36,000 in the US yearly, such a supervirus might kill millions as medical facilities and personnel become overwhelmed, vaccines and antivirals are depleted and social order is stressed.

Symptoms and Signs

Similar to seasonal flu, but more severe: fever, chills, headache, cough, sore throat, runny nose, aches and fatigue. Eventually: pneumonia, pulmonary failure and death.

Treatment

Treatment will depend on the strain and the circumstances. Antivirals like Tamiflu® can be effective and the US government has a supply of vaccine stockpiled. However, it is likely that the supply of both will be depleted quickly in the outbreak. Prevention and a sound public health policy is the best strategy.

Precautions and Prevention

The enormous reservoir of bird and swine flu virus and the rapid dissemination and contagious potential of airline travel mean that the pandemic may come with blistering speed and ferocity. There are measures that both protect the individual and decrease the risk to all Americans:

• Always get the annual flu shot. You <u>cannot</u> get flu or autism from the vaccine and it protects you from the seasonal flu and lowers both your personal risk and the nation's risk for bird flu or swine flu epidemics.

• Practice correct sneeze etiquette (See The Common Cold).

- Wash hands properly and often (See Hand Washing).

- Don't touch your hands to your face, eyes, nose or mouth.

- Follow public health advisories.

- If traveling abroad, avoid open poultry markets and pig farms. Don't handle birds or bird droppings. Notify your physician if you think you have been exposed to bird or swine flu.

  Go to www.flu.gov for authoritative information and references.

Mononucleosis (Mono)

Infectious mononucleosis or 'mono' is a contagious disease caused by the Epstein-Barr virus (EBV), a herpesvirus. It is transmitted through saliva and close contact; therefore it is often called the 'kissing disease'. Mono can also be contracted by exposure to a cough, sneeze, sharing a drinking glass or toothbrush. Most of us were exposed to the EBV as young children with mild or no symptoms and have developed immunity. However, when EBV infection occurs during early adulthood, the disease is more serious. Once you are infected, the incubation period is 4 to 8 weeks before symptoms appear and symptoms last for 2 to 4 weeks with fatigue lasting several months. EBV has been linked to Chronic Fatigue Syndrome (CFS); fatigue lasting longer than six months may suggest CFS.

Symptoms

- Sore throat and swollen tonsils. Often white patches on tonsils.
- Swollen lymph glands
- Fever
- Fatigue and weakness
- Headache
- Skin rash
- Enlarged, fragile spleen and liver
- Night sweats

Diagnosis

Your doctor will examine you, evaluate your symptoms and order lab tests to confirm the diagnosis. The tests may include an antibody test for EBV called a monospot test, EBV serology, complete blood count and throat culture. However, in the early stages of infection lab tests may be inconclusive.

Treatment

The main treatment of mono is supportive in nature: fluids, bed rest, and medications to treat the symptoms such as Tylenol or Advil for pain or fever. The symptoms may last for several months. Mononucleosis usually causes enlargement of the spleen with an increased risk of rupture and bleeding if you return to vigorous activity too soon. In addition, be aware that you are contagious for months after your infection.

Acute Bronchitis

Acute bronchitis is inflammation of the air passages to the lungs caused by an infection or irritation. Infections are usually viral, rarely bacterial, and may spread from the nose to the lungs. Irritations are environmental: smoke, smog, pollution, and allergens.

Symptoms

The lungs respond first with a dry cough, and then produce yellow or green mucus to trap and remove the irritant or infection. Wheezing, low fever, fatigue, muscle aches, nasal congestion or sore throat may occur.

Treatment

Help the lung cleanse itself. Use a mist humidifier or vaporizer. Stay well hydrated. Take an OTC expectorant such as guaifenesin to thin and aid removal of mucus. Avoid cough suppressants (dextromethorphan) unless you have a <u>dry</u> cough; the key is coughing the mucus out. Take acetaminophen for aches, fever or pain. Hard candy soothes the throat. Since most bronchitis is viral, antibiotics are ineffective and potentially harmful. Symptoms last 2-3 weeks and can be treated at home. Call your physician if you have a prolonged fever greater than 102°F, difficulty breathing, wheezing, shortness of breath, a cough that last more than 2 weeks, blood in your mucus or severe painful coughing. These could be symptoms of pneumonia, a much more serious illness.

Respiratory Infections and Asthma

Bronchitis, sinus infections, influenza or colds can trigger an asthmatic attack. Asthma symptoms include wheezing, coughing and difficulty breathing. Cough Variant Asthma: signs are coughing with no mucus or fever and can mimic bronchitis however this form of asthma is usually caused by allergies or asthmatic triggers rather than an infection.

Diarrhea, Vomiting and GI Distress

The two most common causes of diarrhea are food poisoning and viral gastroenteritis (stomach flu). They are often hard to differentiate as the symptoms are very similar. Viral gastroenteritis, misnamed 'stomach flu', is unrelated to the influenza (flu) respiratory virus. Food poisoning is caused by foods or beverages contaminated with bacteria, parasites or viruses. Causes can include undercooked meats, contaminated water, unwashed produce, food handlers that do not wash their hands (fecal contamination) or sharing eating utensils with someone who is infected.

Symptoms

• Nausea, vomiting, abdominal cramps and diarrhea.

• Fever, headache, muscle weakness, loss of appetite.

• Symptoms may last for 1 to 10 days.

Treatment

• Slowly replenish fluids with ice chips, clear juices, sports drinks or oral hydration fluid.

• The next step is a bland diet: soda crackers, mashed potatoes, cubed chicken, Jell-O, broth. The BRAT Diet is especially for GI upset: **B**ananas **R**ice **A**pplesauce **T**oast. BRAT foods bind and promote solid stool.

• Advance your diet slowly from bland diet to soft diet (soup, eggs, yogurt). Maintain protein intake.

• Avoid ibuprofen (Advil, Motrin) and aspirin because of its potential for stomach upset. If fever is present, then take acetaminophen (Tylenol).

• Avoid spicy foods, dairy, caffeine, alcohol and fatty foods.

• Use bismuth subsalicylate (Pepto-Bismol) for relief of diarrhea. Note: Your tongue and stool may have a black color due to the bismuth.

• Take your temperature.

• Keep daily record of the amount of fluid you take in, the medicine you take (so you do not exceed maximum recommended amount) and your temperature.

• Stool sample can be used to test for bacteria, parasites or viral gastroenteritis. Antibiotics may be prescribed for a bacterial infection.

• Call your doctor or go to urgent care facility if you have blood in your stool or vomit, persistent vomiting for more than a day, persistent abdominal pain, if you are dehydrated or if the diarrhea lasts longer than 3 days. Dehydration can be a serious complication that may require hospitalization and intravenous fluid therapy.

• Call your PCP for advice and treatment.

Prevention

• See section on Contagious Diseases.

• Wash your hands, avoid contact with contaminated surfaces, do not share utensils, and do not eat undercooked or raw meat, especially ground beef and chicken. Thaw meat in the refrigerator, never on the counter or in hot water.

• Avoid buffet meals or any publicly exposed food displays.

• Choose popular restaurants; food turnover is faster so there is less spoilage.

• Wash your produce.

Constipation

Constipation is defined as: hard stools, straining, incomplete emptying or three days without a bowel movement. Fortunately, constipation is preventable. Sporadic constipation is normal but chronic constipation has serious health risks including hemorrhoids, bowel disease, diverticulosis, diverticulitis and perhaps even the #2 killer of Americans, colon cancer. All these diseases are thought to be caused by retaining waste and carcinogens, poor bowel health and increased abdominal pressure during valsalva (holding your breath and straining).

Common Causes

Usually constipation is caused by diet: inadequate fluids or fiber, highly processed foods, change in diet and dairy foods. Narcotics, iron supplements, antidepressants, antacids and other drugs can cause constipation. Depression, stress and a lack of exercise are contributing factors.

Laxative Types

Bulk Forming: Complex natural carbohydrates like Metamucil and Citrucel absorb water, making stool larger and softer. Regular use is safe, and in some patients, highly recommended. Good hydration is essential. Advance slowly, as bloating and gas may occur.

Stool Softeners: Docusate lubricates and softens stool, making it easier to pass. Need good hydration. Use for one week only.

Osmotic Agents: Lactulose, sorbitol and other nonabsorbable sugars act by drawing water into the colon and softening stool. Consult MD before use.

Stimulants/Irritants: Castor oil and others. These act by irritating the intestinal lining, and frequent use can cause dependency and/or alter the tone of the bowel wall. Frequent use is not advised. Consult MD.

Prevention

There is epidemiological evidence that healthy, high fiber diets can decrease risk of bowel disease including colon polyps and cancer. Fresh fruits, vegetables, bran, oatmeal and good fluid intake plus exercise vastly improve symptoms and bowel health. Dietary changes may be the miracle cure.

Pearls

- Keys: Regular exercise, a healthy high fiber diet and good hydration.
- Use coffee/tea to stimulate the gastrocolic reflex (colon contractions after food/drink enters an empty stomach). Get in a daily rhythm by eating a healthy oatmeal/bran breakfast with coffee and then having a bowel movement, followed by your morning shower. This bowel routine improves personal hygiene, reduces flatulence and may lower your risk of colon cancer.

Call your doctor if condition persists or worsens.

Fever

Fever is a temperature above 100.4°F caused by infection or illness, as opposed to heat injury, which is elevated T° due to external causes (see Heat Injury). They both present with high T°, but are very different in etiology and treatment.

Fever is often feared as a dangerous condition that must be treated. In truth, fever is not a disease; it is a healthy natural response to infection. Fever increases blood flow, activates enzymes and the immune system and kills heat sensitive bacteria and viruses. All the body's defenses work better at a higher temperature. The fever will usually subside in 2-3 days as the infection is controlled.

There are many fever myths. These are the facts: Body T° fluctuates constantly with an average of 98.6°F; most fevers won't cause brain damage (only T° over 107.6°F causes brain damage) and mild fevers do not need to be lowered.

Thermometers

Dispose properly of old glass mercury thermometers, they are poisonous. Digital thermometers are accurate and safer. Oral or axillary T° is fine. Thermometer strips should only be used for axillary T°. Ear thermometers are expensive and can be imprecise.

The best choice is an oral, digital thermometer.

Treatment of Fever

Healthy adults can tolerate fevers of up to 104°F. Physicians do not look at just the T°; they look at the whole patient. If uncomfortable with high fever (102-104°F), fever should be treated with:

• OTC antipyretics (acetaminophen, NSAIDs).

• Tepid water bath (never ice) or sponging with water (never alcohol).

• Maintain good hydration.

• Liquid diet if awake and stable.

Seek medical advice in cases of prolonged fever, fever in a compromised adult, or if symptoms of serious illness occur.

Steps For Advancing Diet When Sick

During a cold, flu, fever or any illness or surgery you must stay adequately hydrated and nourished. You lose fluid and electrolytes with fevers, sweats, vomiting and diarrhea, and your metabolism is elevated which increases your need for fuel. Failure to stay hydrated and nourished can worsen your condition and prolong the illness. Advancing your diet should be done slowly, going to the next step as tolerated (without nausea or vomiting) until you are back to normal.

Feed a Fever, Starve a Cold = MYTH

This nonsense dates back to the 1500s when physicians bled patients and wise men knew the world was flat. It is probably best to disregard this old wives' tale. You need nutrition; feed both a fever and a cold.

Steps for Advancing Diet

1. Sips and Chips: Small sips of tepid water and little ice chips while sitting up soothes the mouth and rehydrates. Go slow, gradually increasing volume.

2. Electrolyte Replacement: Vomiting, diarrhea and sweating deplete fluid and electrolytes. Potassium, sodium, calcium, zinc are all critical to cell function. Drink a low calorie sports drink. Pedialyte® is excellent. Avoid artificially sweetened drinks and high fructose corn syrup.

3. Clear Liquids: Chicken soup with garlic, chicken broth, gelatin, apple juice, sports drinks with protein. <u>Never Drink</u>: tea, cola, coffee, soft drinks, caffeine drinks. These are diuretics and will further deplete fluids and electrolytes.

4. Full Liquids: Full bodied soups, yogurt, pureed foods. Soft foods may be put in a blender and liquefied. Fruit smoothies. Sports gels. Go slow. These foods will stimulate the bowels; if diarrhea or nausea occurs, go back to clear liquids.

5. Bland Diet: Soda crackers. Mashed potatoes. Cubed chicken. The BRAT Diet is especially for GI upset: **B**ananas **R**ice **A**pplesauce **T**oast. BRAT foods bind and promote solid stool.

6. Finally, gradually return to a regular diet including protein, vegetables, grains and fruits. Include flavonoids and Vitamin C, both found in

grapefruit, oranges, lemons and limes, to boost the immune system and speed recovery. Vitamin B6 and B12 are immune boosters as are phytochemicals found in fruits and vegetables. Take a multivitamin.

Post-operatively, surgeons advance patients' diets slowly, listening to bowel sounds and evaluating vital signs. At home, you have to go slowly using your own judgment. If nausea, vomiting or diarrhea recurs, slow down, go back one step and start again. The duration of each stage will depend upon the severity of your illness and your general health, but a rule of thumb, for a mild to moderate GI flu, you can use 6-8 hours per stage, assuming that there is no relapse or increase of symptoms. More severe illnesses may take longer. Fortunately, many of the new sports drinks and sports gels have protein, carbs, vitamins and nutrients in dense, easily absorbed form.

Homemade Sports Drink and Resuscitation Formula

There are a wide variety of commercially available sports and endurance drinks tailored to many specific needs. Studies in sports physiology show that oral fluid uptake is accelerated by using a formula consisting of water, sugar and electrolytes. These formulas rehydrate more rapidly than pure water and also restore energy and replace lost sodium, potassium and other electrolytes, thereby improving muscle and nerve conduction. An expedient formula is simple, easily made at home and can be used for fluid replacement after exercise or illness.

Formula

32 ounces of tap or bottled water

1/4 cup sugar

1/4 teaspoon salt

1 tablespoon of lemon or lime juice or 1/2 cup fruit juice

Mix well and refrigerate

Approximate Volume Measurements and Conversions

1 teaspoon = 5 milliliters

3 teaspoons = 1 tablespoon = 15 milliliters

16 tablespoons = 1 cup

1 cup = 8 ounces = 250 milliliters

2 cups = 1 pint = 16 ounces = 500 milliliters

4 cups = 1 quart = 32 ounces = 1 liter

4 quarts = 1 gallon = 128 ounces = 4 liters

Dorm/Apartment Medical Kit

These are items that you should have available to avoid a late night trip to the drugstore or doctor.

First Aid Kit (available at drugstores or outdoor recreation stores) with instruction booklet. To this kit add:

• Your prescription medicines.

• Epi-pen (for life threatening allergies if prescribed by doctor).

• Analgesics (acetaminophen, aspirin or ibuprofen).

• Daytime and nighttime cold medicine.

• Anti-diarrheal (Pepto-Bismol).

• Anti-fungal (Monistat).

• Anti-histamine (Benadryl).

• Topical anti-histamine cream (Benadryl/diphenhydramine)

• Antibiotic ointment (Bacitracin).

• Hydrocortisone cream.

• Eye care items (normal saline drops).

• Magnifying glasses.

• Tweezers, tick remover and safety pin.

• Assorted Band-Aids®.

• Moleskin (for blisters).

• Scissors, knife and sterile needles.

• Antibacterial soap.

• Alcohol swabs packets (individually wrapped).

• Antiseptic wipes (individually wrapped).

• Gauze (various sizes).

• Antiseptic (for intact skin only).

• J&J Band-Aid® Hurt-Free Antiseptic Wash (for open wounds).

• Ace Bandages.

• Cloth tape.

• Duct tape.

- Disposable non-sterile exam gloves.

- Instant ice pack.

- Digital thermometer.

- Medicine cup.

- Save-A-Tooth.

www.mayoclinic.com has an outstanding section on First Aid

Water and Dehydration

- Water makes up 60% of our body by weight and is essential to our body's normal function.
- You lose water through sweating, breathing, excreting and urinating. If you lose more than you take in you become dehydrated.
- To maintain a normal level of water, adult males should consume 3 liters of fluid per day and adult females 2.2 liters of fluid per day. Since water is present in our food, we will obtain some of our water from eating but most is obtained by drinking.
- The "8 x 8" rule suggests that you drink eight 8 ounce glasses of water per day or 1.9 liters per day as a general guideline.
- Are you drinking enough water? You can monitor your hydration by observing your urine output; it should be clear (yellow, not dark) and copious (about 1.5 liters per day).

Dehydration

- Failure to stay hydrated during hot summer days, athletic activities, hikes, working outside or any exertion can lead to dehydration. Dehydration, if left untreated, can lead to heat exhaustion and even heatstroke.
- Symptoms include thirst, dark urine or decreased urine output, weakness, headache, and confusion.
- If you are thirsty, you are in early dehydration.
- Drink throughout the day, and maintain good urine output. Your urine should be "clear and copious".
- Treatment of dehydration is to rest in a cool area and drink water or sports drink slowly until symptoms subside.

Prevention

- Hydrate before, during and after activity and in hot weather conditions even when activity level is low. Avoid coffee, tea, caffeine, cola and alcohol. Wear light, loose, moisture wicking clothing.

Bottled Water vs. Tap Water

Perhaps the greatest marketing genius of all time is the one who convinced us that we should drink bottled water at $7 per gallon, more than the price of gasoline. Recent evidence indicates that bottled water may be costly in terms of environmental impact as well, all with no real advantage over tap water. The reality is that most bottled water, despite panoramic mountains or glacier images on the label, is just reprocessed municipal tap water.

- Blind taste tests show that bottled water and tap water are roughly equivalent in flavor.

- Lab analysis of tap vs. bottled water shows no significant difference in chemical, bacteria or contaminant levels. And while the EPA requires testing of tap water for the intestinal parasites cryptosporidium and giardia, there are no such testing requirements for bottled water.

- Cost of bottled water is from 500 to 25,000 times greater than tap water.

- Environmental impact of the plastic water bottles is substantial, with 2 million tons of empty bottles in landfills yearly.

- Essential minerals, such as enamel hardening fluoride, may be missing from bottled water. This lack of fluoride may result in dental decay.

- "Enhanced Water": Sports waters, fitness waters, energy waters and other super waters offer no significant health advantages, and may contain excess sugar and unwanted calories. Take a daily multivitamin instead.

Water is water. We take for granted the seemingly limitless supply of clean, healthy tap water at our fingertips, for about a penny per gallon. If taste or residual chlorine is an issue, using water filters and citrus wedges will improve palatability of municipal tap water. For times when we need convenience and portability, a reusable stainless steel water bottle stays cold better than plastic, has no BPA, costs less in the long run and protects the environment. There are a few situations when bottled water is recommended: foreign travel, airline travel or natural disasters where the water supply is compromised. All other times, tap water is preferable, cheaper and healthier.

Heat Cramps, Heat Exhaustion and Heat Stroke

An elevated T° caused by extreme heat is different from fever due to infection. Heat overwhelming the body's ability to stay cool is a life threatening medical emergency. The three following conditions are a result of heat and dehydration.

Heat Cramps

Heat cramps are rare except in prolonged exertion in hot environments without replacement of water and electrolytes. Symptoms are strong, painful contractions of muscles. Treatment is replacement of salts with sports drinks and rehydration.

Heat Exhaustion

Heat exhaustion occurs on hot days, often with dehydration. The body's ability to keep cool is beginning to fail. Symptoms: pale, clammy skin, nausea/vomiting, weakness, fainting, headache and muscle cramps. Signs: Dark urine, rapid heart rate, low blood pressure. T° up to 104°F.

Treatment: Get out of the heat, apply wet cold compresses, take water/sports drink and salty foods slowly and remove unnecessary clothing. If symptoms persist, call 911.

Heatstroke

Heat exhaustion may progress to heatstroke, a life threatening condition. Heatstroke occurs as core temperature exceeds 105° and brain damage begins at 107.6° as the body's regulatory system fails. Death may occur if not treated promptly. Symptoms and Signs: hot flushed and dry skin, mental confusion, seizures, coma and rapid heart and respiratory rates.

<u>Call 911 immediately.</u>
<u>DO NOT: Use ice bath or give aspirin, acetaminophen, etc. to reduce fever.</u>

Treatment: Cool ASAP with cold compresses, air conditioning or immersion in cool water. Ice packs to armpits and groin. Remove clothing; fan and mist. Rehydration with water/sports drink if victim lucid. Establish communication with 911 for assistance.

Headache (HA)

Headaches are extremely common but rarely serious. They occur by themselves and as a secondary symptom with many other illnesses, allergies and environmental stress. There are three main types of headaches:

Tension Headaches/Stress Headaches

This HA is described as having a metal band around the head, gradually tightening. Pain is mild to moderate, and may eventually involve the entire head. There are no other symptoms and activity does not exacerbate the pain. Treatment is OTC analgesics.

Migraine Headaches

Migraine headaches are not completely understood. They seem to be hereditary, related to the arteries to the brain, stress and estrogen levels. The pain is moderate to severe and can be debilitating. Pain is throbbing, usually on one side, and characteristically aggravated by light, noise and activity. Often there is an aura that precedes the attack and an unusual mental state that follows afterward. These can be visual or olfactory hallucinations, flashing lights, blind spots or strange smells, but almost any neurological symptom could occur. Treatment is complex and personalized to the patient, and may require a thorough evaluation by a neurologist and prescription medications.

Cluster Headaches

Occurring in clusters lasting 4-8 weeks, these headaches are rare. They tend to begin in or around the eye or temple, then spread to one side of the head. Pain is severe, unrelenting and very intense, often driving the patient to episodes of head banging. Treatment may require prescription medication.

Medical Alert: Dangerous Headaches

The vast majority of headaches are benign and self limiting, but some represent warning signs of a serious condition and require prompt medical treatment. Headaches that change character or pattern, become more painful or frequent, wake you from sleep, are associated with weakness, fainting or visual changes, sensory changes or motor changes, occur after head or neck trauma or are accompanied by neck stiffness should be evaluated by a physician promptly.

Meningitis

Meningitis is the inflammation or infection of the meninges, the membrane surrounding the brain and spinal cord. It is most often caused by a bacterial or viral infection, and because 30% of all cases involve young adults, it is a health concern for college students. There are about 3,000 cases per year with approximately 300 deaths per year. Crowded living conditions and the communal living in dormitories or fraternity and sorority houses make college students more likely to acquire the disease.

Symptoms

- Fever

- Nausea and vomiting

- Severe headache

- Stiff neck

- Altered mental status or confusion

- Sensitivity to light (photophobia)

- Tachycardia (fast heart rate)

- Drowsiness

- Skin rash

Meningitis is a medical emergency and you should go to the student health clinic or ER immediately. Your doctor may take a blood culture, CT scan of the head and a cerebrospinal fluid (CSF) sample (spinal tap) for culture and analysis.

Treatment

If you are diagnosed with bacterial meningitis your doctor will prescribe antibiotics and may admit you to the hospital for intravenous fluids and support. Complications of bacterial meningitis include brain injury, hearing loss, paralysis, blindness, seizures and death. Viral meningitis is less severe and rarely fatal; it usually runs a course of 7-10 days with full recovery.

Prevention

Since meningitis is a contagious disease, one can prevent contracting or spreading meningitis with good hygiene, washing your hands, good nutrition and covering your mouth when coughing or sneezing. It is also recommended and sometimes required by colleges that incoming students obtain immunizations to prevent meningitis.

Fainting (Syncope)

Fainting or syncope is the brief loss of consciousness that occurs because of lack of blood flow to the brain. Usually fainting is short lived and the person regains consciousness within a few minutes. There are three phases of syncope: pre-syncope, syncope and recovery. In the pre-syncope phase, the person will have a symptom of lightheadedness followed by syncope or unconsciousness and usually recovery occurs within minutes with a return to consciousness.

Causes

- Dehydration, low blood sugar (hypoglycemia).

- Seizures, heart problems, diabetes, some medications.

- Panic attack or stress. In this case, we faint because fear or anxiety has initiated the "fight or flight" response which sends blood to our large muscle groups (legs). However, if we don't fight or flee, the pooling of blood in the legs starves the brain of oxygen, causing syncope. Movement of our legs during this process re-circulates the blood flow.

Symptoms

- Pre-syncope symptoms include nausea, lightheadedness, sweating, pale skin color, increased heart rate.

- Syncope symptoms include low blood pressure and slow heart rate, cold extremities, visual disturbances, loss of consciousness.

Treatment

- Place patient flat on their back with legs and feet up.

- Check for consciousness.

- Begin CAB. Circulation-Airway-Breathing. Call 911.

- Give oxygen if available.

- Use ammonia stimulant if available.

- Apply cold compress to forehead or neck.

- Relax and reassure patient.

- Once stable, consult a physician for a full evaluation.

Prevention

- Maintain good hydration and eat a healthy diet.

- Control anxiety and know when you are stressed.

- If you feel that you are going to faint, lie down and raise your legs and feet. Use a bicycle motion to move pooled blood to heart and brain.

Burns

There are three classifications of burns: 1st, 2nd and 3rd degree burns.

First degree burns are superficial, when only the outer layer, or epidermis, of skin is burned. The skin is red and tender with mild pain. Treat with cool water and cool wet compresses.

Second degree burns have burned through the outer layer of skin and into the dermis or second layer. A blister forms and the site is red, swollen and splotchy with severe pain. Treatment of the second degree burn includes:

- Cool the burn with cool running water or wet cold compresses.
- Cover with loose, sterile gauze.
- Take Advil or Tylenol for pain.
- <u>Do not use ice</u>, as it will cause further damage.
- <u>Do not apply lotions, jellies, butter or ointments</u> to burn. This will delay healing or cause infection.
- <u>Do not break blisters,</u> as they are a natural protective mechanism and the site will become susceptible to infection.
- Watch for infection or worsening condition. Seek medical attention.
- Avoid re-injury or sunburn in area of burn or pigmentation will occur.

Third degree burns are the most severe and occur with thermal injury to deeper tissues including muscle, fat and nerve. This is life threatening.

- Remove person from source of burn.
- Call 911.
- <u>Do not remove clothing</u> that is burnt.
- <u>Do not immerse extensive burns</u> into cool water, as shock may occur.
- Cover burnt area with clean towel or sheets.
- Begin CAB of CPR and treat for shock as indicated.

Poisoning

Poisoning is the second leading cause of injury related deaths, with almost a million ER visits and 33,000 deaths annually. Only motor vehicle accidents are more lethal. While it is commonly believed that poisonings primarily occur in children, the reality is that most fatalities are in adults, and 70% are accidental.

Causes of Poisoning

- Medications: pain, heart, sleep, OTC medications. Never put medications in old/different bottles.

- Household chemicals: drain cleaners, toilet bowl cleaners, detergents, insecticides, lime and rust removers, oven cleaners, lighter fluid.

- Automotive chemicals: antifreeze, windshield fluid, solvents.

- Cosmetics: nail polish removers, nail polish, perfume, mouthwash.

- Mixing medications and alcohol.

Symptoms and Signs

There is no typical presentation for poisonings. Symptoms vary widely, depending upon the poison; however nausea, vomiting, pain, difficulty breathing or change in skin color may be seen. Call the National Poison Control Center immediately if poisoning is suspected.

Treatment of Poisoning

Contact the National Poison Control Center immediately.

800.222.1222

Do not induce vomiting or use syrup of ipecac.
Do not give activated charcoal.

Keep the National Poison Control Center number by the phone. Remain calm and give them as much information as you can, including any drugs, drug bottles, household chemicals or other evidence you suspect may be related to the poisoning. They will provide directions for appropriate home treatment or advise that you go to the hospital if necessary. The vast majority of poisonings do not require medical intervention, and are treated successfully at home.

The Sun, Sunburn and Tanning Salons

Skin cancer rates are skyrocketing, and are related to sun exposure. Sunburn and tanning is skin damage from overexposure to UVA and UVB rays. UV radiation destroys collagen and elastin causing wrinkles, and damages cellular DNA and weakens the immune system, causing skin cancer. Repeated sunburn amplifies these effects. UV eye exposure leads to cataracts and macular degeneration. There is no "healthy tan" or "safe tan". Tanned or burned skin is damaged skin.

Medical Alert: Tanning Salons

Never use tanning salons. Evidence suggests that they are far more dangerous than the sun due to higher UVA exposure than natural sunlight and increased intensity. Long wavelength UVA penetrates deeper than UVB, causing less burn but greater tissue damage. The American Academy of Dermatology states: "The use of indoor tanning beds before the age of 35 has been associated with a significant increase in the risk of melanoma, the deadliest form of skin cancer."

Prevention

- Apply sunscreen with SPF of 15 or higher to all exposed skin. Only use sunscreens that block UVA and UVB. Reapply often.

- Use a quality makeup base with SPF 15.

- Wear clothing with high SPF (tight weave). Cotton has an SPF of 7, Polyester of 35 and denim is 1700.

- Wear a hat with a wide and full brim or neck cape (not baseball caps which have no ear coverage) for face/head/ear/neck coverage.

- Sit in the shade.

- Avoid sun between 10AM and 3PM when the sun is the strongest.

- Never go to tanning salons. Ever.

- If you want a tan, use self tanning lotions or spray-on tan.

- Wear sunglasses when outside to protect your eyes from UV light. Use sunglasses that have UVA and UVB protection.

Treatment

- If you have sunburn, immediately get out of the sun.
- Soak area in cool water to lower temperature of skin, and reduce inflammation and pain.
- Sunburns will depress your immune system for 3 days. Stay healthy.
- Take ibuprofen to reduce inflammation and pain.
- Drink green tea and eat antioxidant foods.
- Moisturize and use topical antioxidants such as Vit E and green tea extract.
- Avoid topical anesthetics. Using topical anesthetics on open wounds like sunburn may increase sensitivity and allergic reactions.
- Avoid repeat exposure.

Nosebleeds

The nose has a rich blood supply to warm, humidify and filter the air we breathe. Environmental stress on the nose is high and occasional nosebleeds are common. These minor bleeds are from one side only, near the tip of the nose, and are easily treated at home. A nosebleed from trauma is often a fracture.

Medical Alert: Traumatic Nosebleed

Trauma resulting in a nosebleed should be evaluated and treated promptly. Seek medical attention immediately.

Causes

Arteries in the nose are only covered with thin mucosa and are fragile. The main causes of bleeds are repetitive irritation (picking) or harsh dry air. Smoke, fumes, colds and flu, allergies and high altitude are factors. Drugs like aspirin, NSAIDs, nasal decongestant or steroid sprays, ginko, methamphetamine or cocaine can cause nosebleeds.

Treatment

The bleeding is usually in the septum, the structure dividing the two nasal cavities. By applying pressure to the nose, from the bones above all the way down to the tip, bleeding can be controlled.

- Apply pressure as soon as you notice bleeding. If bleeding has gone on for a while, gently blow out clots and blood, and then apply pressure.

- Spit out blood. Do not swallow blood, this may cause vomiting.

- Sit upright, tilt head forward. Breathe through your mouth only.

- Thumb on one side, two fingers on the other, grip between the eyes and slide down the bony nose until you have the entire soft part of the nose firmly gripped.

- Apply pressure for 15 minutes, by the clock.

- Release gently, check for bleeding. If bleeding continues, repeat for another 15 minutes, by the clock.

- Ice or frozen pea pack to the bridge of the nose helps.

- Rest quietly. Sleep elevated on two pillows.

- Do not blow nose for 2 days. No aspirin, NSAIDs or herbal supplements.
- If bleeding persists, seek medical care.

Prevention

Preventive measures include no nose picking, good hydration and applying Vaseline inside nose during dry months, using humidifiers and saline nasal sprays. Seek medical care if bleeds occur frequently.

Sprains and Strains

Sprains and strains are very common musculoskeletal injuries and usually can be treated at home. A sprain is damage to ligaments surrounding and supporting a joint. A strain is damage to muscle fibers or tendons. Often sports related, they are caused by poor footwear, not warming up, uneven surfaces, falls, and twisting. They are discussed together because they are similar in many ways, and prevention is the best cure.

Symptoms and Signs

Sprain: pain, swelling, bruising, pops, joint stiffness.

Strain: pain, swelling, spasm, muscle stiffness.

Treatment: *PRICE*

Protection: Cease the sport/activity. Do not use the injured area. Splint or sling.

Rest: Do not use the injured area, especially in first 48-72 hrs.

Ice: Cold packs will decrease pain, swelling and inflammation in first 48 hrs. Apply the pack for 10 minutes on, then 20-30 minutes off. Never place ice pack directly on your skin; use a washcloth or towel between pack and skin.

Compression: *Gently* wrap the area with elastic bandage to reduce swelling.

Elevation: Keep area above level of heart as much as possible, and at night. This will decrease swelling, inflammation and pain. Elevate on pillows.

Rehab and recovery: aspirin, ibuprofen or acetaminophen for pain and inflammation. Gradually increase motion. Pain is the red flag to slow down or stop.

Consult physician if you suspect fracture, can't walk, can't move the joint, have numbness, deformity, redness, joint is unstable, muscle will not function or conditions get worse with time.

Prevention

Proper gear: Wear the right shoes for the sport. Use gel insoles to cushion impacts. A good shoe and sole should stabilize the ankle. Specific braces or wraps help stabilize joints. Always warm up to stretch ligaments and muscles that tighten when unused. Condition yourself for your sport slowly. Avoid new and unfamiliar sports until conditioned. Cool down after a workout. Never exercise when fatigued. This dramatically increases risk of injury. Rest before you become tired.

Medical Alert: Elastic Wraps

Learn how to properly wrap. If done incorrectly, a wrap will aggravate the injury and possibly cause severe or life threatening conditions such as blood clots or gangrene. Go to www.webMD.com for specific tutorials.

The Basics:

Elevate the limb to allow blood to drain. Start wrap farthest from heart and gently wrap toward heart. Remove if pain increases, redness, throbbing, skin blanching, numbness, swelling or no pulse below wrap or shifting of the wrap. Never drink alcohol or use drugs, including painkillers, with wrap on incorrectly or tightly. Check the wrap frequently.

Blisters

Blisters are caused by friction or heat related burns. Trauma causes fluid formation, sometimes with blood, beneath the skin. Because this fluid is often sterile, it is usually best not to open blisters unless they are on the hands, feet, infected or painful. The fluid and intact blister promote rapid healing.

For small blisters or non-painful blisters, no treatment is required.

For larger painful blisters or blisters on the hands or feet, use the following technique:

• Wash hands, wear gloves, clean blister with disinfectant soap or solution.

• Sterilize the end of a needle with heat (until red, then allow to cool) or by soaking in disinfectant soap for 5 minutes.

• Puncture at the base of blister with needle, releasing fluid. Keep overlying skin intact.

• Apply antibiotic ointment and dress with moleskin that has a hole in the middle the size of the blister. Put the hole over the blister so that the moleskin protects the area around the blister, leaving the blister untouched.

• Change the dressing daily and check for infection.

Prevention

Prevent blisters by keeping well hydrated, thus reducing friction. Use gloves when using tools or using hands with repetitive motion. Select shoes that fit properly and have ½ inch of space between the end of your toes and the shoe. Choose shoes that breathe well and that do not slip off your foot. Choose soft fabric socks that wick moisture away from foot, not cotton due to its moisture absorbent quality. Use a moleskin or Blister Block™ when you feel a "hot spot" or developing blister.

Loud Music and Loud Noises

Anyone who has studied the anatomy of the middle and inner ear is struck with its intricate delicacy and beauty. Sound waves are captured and funneled through the ear canal, amplified by three tiny bones in the middle ear, turned into fluid waves in the inner ear and finally translated into electrical energy to transmit to the brain. We have eyelids to protect the eyes, but nothing protects the fragile inner ear. And while it is often considered silly to use ear protection, the resultant poor hearing is cause for ridicule. The tragedy is that outstanding hearing protection is readily available, cheap and disposable: soft foam earplugs.

Noise damages the ear, and our world is full of noise: occupational noise in construction, manufacturing, shops and garages, farming; recreational noise from motorcycles, ATVs, snowmobiles, shooting, music, rock concerts; daily life noise from traffic, sirens, jet engines; personal noise from hair dryers, vacuum cleaners, lawn mowers, blenders, small appliances and especially mp3/iPod earbuds. There are two mechanisms of hearing injury: sustained 80db+ noise causing slow damage and sudden 100db+ noise causing immediate permanent damage. The effects are cumulative.

Keep a set of earplugs in your car or purse. Use them any time there may be harmful noise levels. Keep a quality ear muff headset in the house for yard work, vacuuming and using tools. Protect yourself. Hearing damage is irreversible and irreparable.

How to Insert Foam Earplugs

- Roll plug into a cylinder between thumb and forefinger.
- With opposite hand, reach over head and pull ear up and back.
- Gently insert plug and allow to expand in ear canal.
- If sound is not dampened, reinsert properly.
- Remove slowly and gently.

HEAROS has a wide line of soft comfortable ear protection for many applications, and will give you a free sample at www.hearos.com.

Hypothermia

Hypothermia is a life threatening medical emergency where core temperature drops and organs shut down. It is most often seen in extreme cold, wind, being in water or on cold ground and with alcohol/drugs. Correct diagnosis is critical to survival.

Symptoms and Signs

Shivering, confusion, lethargy, coma. Dangerous because signs come on gradually, and the victim may not realize it. As core temperature drops, heart and brain function slows and eventually stops.

Treatment

The goal is to rewarm core T°. Assess closely: Pulse and respiratory rates may be faint and very slow. Do CPR if you are trained and competent. The heart is fragile; undue compressions may cause death. Rescue breathing will warm core.

• Handle gently. Do not rub or massage or exercise.

• Get to warm, dry place.

• Remove wet clothing, shoes, jewelry by cutting if necessary.

• Dry the body gently and cover and insulate from the ground and wind.

• Strip and share body heat with skin contact, bundled in blankets.

• Warm the core: Use warm compresses/towels and apply to neck, groin, underarms, and chest. This warms the arterial blood and core. Never use direct heat.

• Never apply warmth to extremities, arms, legs as this may release pooled cold acidic blood and cause cardiac arrest. Treat frostbite later.

• As patient improves, give warm fluids (no alcohol/caffeine/tea)

• Do not give up. They can come back. The dictum is: "Not dead until warm and dead."

Frostbite

Frostbite is injury to the skin and deep tissues from exposure to the cold. It is seen in winter sports and in car accidents or stranded vehicles. Alcohol and drug abuse are factors. Like burns, it is classified in degrees of severity, and if mild can resolve fully. In severe cases, gangrene and amputation follows. Patient assessment is critical, as incorrect first aid may actually worsen the outcome.

Medical Alert: See Hypothermia

In any cold related emergency, first determine if hypothermia exists. Hypothermia must be treated first by raising the core T° of the victim. Warming the extremities in a hypothermic patient can be fatal.

Symptoms

Frostbite affects the extremities first: hands, feet, nose, ears. Tingling will be followed by a wooden feeling. Skin will be pale, hard and numb.

Treatment

Treatment depends on the situation and availability of medical care:

- If medical care is available: Call 911, keep warm, transport to ER.

- If medical care is not available but you have stable shelter and warmth: Rewarm gently in <u>warm</u> water (104-107°) or use warm compresses. Never use hot water or direct heat on frostbite. Circulate water and reapply warm compresses until skin is soft and sensate.

- If medical care is not available, and you cannot get out of the cold: Wrap patient, keep core warm. Do not attempt extremity rewarming. If rewarmed, and refreezing occurs, damage may be irreversible. Wait until situation is stable to rewarm.

Emergency Treatment of Frostbite

Move gently. Remove constricting, wet clothing or jewelry.
Loosen boots. Dry the patient. Separate fingers and toes with dressings.
Keep patient hydrated with warm drinks.

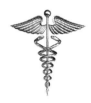

Proper Treatment is Critical

- Never rewarm if there is possibility of further cold exposure; refreezing amplifies the tissue damage.

- Never use direct heat (fire, heat pad, radiator, hair dryer).

- Never massage or rub frostbitten areas.

- Never give alcohol or caffeine/drugs or smoke or use tobacco.

- Never walk on frostbitten feet.

Prevention of Cold Injuries

All cold injury is preventable. Use the buddy system. Dress for the worst possible weather you might encounter. Use layers that can be added or removed to regulate heat loss:

- Base layer: polypropylene wicking underwear and socks.

- Insulating layer: wool/fleece garments and wool socks.

- Top layer: Gore-Tex® windproof/waterproof breathable fabrics.

Wear mittens instead of gloves; mittens keep fingers warmer by minimizing heat loss. Buy high performance clothing and gear. www.rei.com.

Keep in your car: Emergency/survival pack with space blanket, towels, food, water, heat packs and appropriate gear.

Be prepared.

Traumatic Brain Injury (TBI)

TBI has become more prevalent as we create high speed, extreme sports. The cranium evolved to protect the brain from impact resulting from normal locomotion (walking, running), not from biking, skiing, rollerblading, etc. Sports related TBI is increasing, with over 3 million concussions yearly. Concussions are head injuries without visible tissue damage, and despite helmets, are increasing in frequency in football and other contact sports. For anything faster than running, wear a helmet. Use the helmet specific for your sport, properly fit and adjusted to your head. Your brain is precious.

The human brain is encased in heavy, double layered bone. Within the skull, the brain floats in a cushioning bath of cerebrospinal fluid (CSF). Injury to the brain occurs when the head rapidly decelerates, rotates violently or is struck with a hard object. The rebound impact of the brain against the inner wall of the skull can be more harmful than the blow itself. Brain injury can be immediate or delayed. In many cases, the victim seems fine until hours or days later when rising pressure within the skull crushes the brain.

In any trauma with neck injury, mental changes or loss of consciousness, immediate medical treatment is required. Call 911. Never try to move or reposition a victim with a neck or spinal injury.

Check the scalp thoroughly for swelling, cuts or bruises that can be hidden by the hair. Clean any minor cuts and bandage lightly. Seek medical care if indicated. Continuous monitoring of the victim is critical. The first signs of TBI may be subtle mental changes, therefore the patient must be watched carefully. Subdural hematomas can take days, even weeks to develop. Give no alcohol or narcotics, as they mask symptoms. Use only a mild OTC analgesic. Question the victim every few hours to evaluate mental status: What is your name? What day is today? Where are you now? Who is the current US President?

Red Flags: unequal pupils, visual changes, confusion, lethargy, memory loss, nausea, vomiting, bleeding, severe headache, stiff neck, slurred speech, loss of consciousness, motor weakness or paralysis, worsening of symptoms. This is only a partial list of danger signs; if you see these or any unusual changes seek immediate medical treatment. You can't 'shake off' a concussion.

Evaluation of TBI is complex and beyond the scope of this book.

Consult a medical professional in all cases of TBI.

The dangers of TBI cannot be overstated. Impairment, disability or death can result from TBI. Prompt medical attention is critical. Call 911, your PCP or ER for assistance if you see any of the red flags, or suspect TBI.

Depression

Depression is a part of life; it touches all of us now and then, with women affected twice as often as men. Usually, it passes with time. Depression may be exogenous (from outside) as in life changes, death in the family, stress at work or relationship problems. Depression may also be endogenous (from within) as in cases of medical illness, endocrine disorders or abnormal levels of neurotransmitters. While the exact cause and mechanism of depression is not completely understood, there are factors that are implicated: alcohol or drug use, certain medications, heredity, chronic pain and some diseases, e.g. hypothyroidism.

Unfortunately, college students are particularly vulnerable to depression because they are removed from their familiar home surroundings and family support systems and face doubt and uncertainty about their academic and social success, their future and career opportunities. These factors, and a constantly changing life and peer pressure, increase the risk of depression in college students.

Symptoms

The symptoms are classic: sadness, anger, frustration. Profound feelings of inadequacy, helplessness, guilt or self-hatred may accompany the physical symptoms of irritability, malaise and fatigue. Weight gain or loss may occur. Poor mental function, inability to concentrate and sleep disorders are common. Anyone showing these symptoms for more than two weeks or anyone whose functioning becomes impaired should seek help. Morbid thoughts or suicidal ideation are an indication that help should be sought immediately.

Treatment

Depression is not a sign of weakness, and you can't just "tough it out". Fortunately, 80% will improve with treatment. The two primary treatments are antidepressant medications and psychotherapy. An evaluation by your PCP may be needed to rule out medication side effects or illness as a cause. Consultation with a psychiatrist, therapy and/or medications may be indicated. Antidepressant medications take time to act, and patients age 18-24 must be monitored closely because suicidal behavior is more common in this group. The prognosis is good; however some people may battle bouts of depression repeatedly through life. Depression may lead to alcohol or drug use, creating and deepening a vicious cycle.

Prevention

Everyone develops a strategy to cope with depression. Avoiding alcohol or drugs, meditating, exercising, immersion in a hobby or pastime, group activities, support groups or a renewed concentration on work or career may help. Exercise may act both as prevention and treatment. Exercise improves self-esteem and elevates endorphins, which are synthesized in the brain and spinal cord, and act to create a feeling of mild euphoria. Even seemingly trivial things can help: planning and structuring your daily routine, taking time to do the things you truly enjoy, deep breathing or bubble baths. If it works, do it.

Get Help

- Act early. Don't wait and allow the sadness to overwhelm you. Talk with your PCP, friends, family, student health service and community outreach resources.

- Remember: You are not alone. Depression is common and treatable.

- Learn the warning signs of depression. If a friend shows signs, help them get treatment. Often depressed people are unable to recognize that they are impaired.

- Call 800.273.TALK for depression counseling and suicide intervention.

- Call 911 if you have any thoughts of suicide, harming yourself or others.

- Call your physician immediately if you hear imaginary voices, have suicidal thoughts, have crying spells, if your medications seem to affect your mood or if your depression is interfering with your work or family life.

- Call 1.800.SUICIDE or 911.

Suicide Prevention Hotline

800.SUICIDE or 911

www.suicidepreventionlifeline.org

Alcohol

Alcohol is the undisputed leader in substance abuse worldwide. The personal, environmental and societal costs far exceed that of heroin or cocaine. Alcohol damages every organ system, and is the only drug from which withdrawal can be fatal. Alcohol abuse is directly tied to violence and traffic fatalities. Alcoholism or alcohol dependence is a strong desire for and physical dependence upon alcohol. College students often practice "binge drinking", a risky form of alcohol abuse. Binge drinking is classified as 5 drinks in a row for males and 4 drinks in a row for females. However, moderation poses little risk to adults and may even be beneficial. What is moderation? For men – two drinks per day and for women – one drink per day.

- Abstaining from alcohol is the best policy. Drinking in moderation is the second best policy. Underage drinking is illegal and unhealthy. If you are under 21, your brain is still developing and alcohol can retard normal growth and maturation, especially in the prefrontal cortex, the area of higher intellectual function.

- Never drink and drive. Always use a designated driver.

- Never drink alone, use the buddy system.

- Remember: Your liver can only metabolize one drink per hour.

- Beware of alcohol masked by sweet mixers or energy drinks.

- Avoid drinking games; you lose control of how much you drink.

- Use a Breathalyzer to assess your blood alcohol content.

- Not all alcohol is created equal. Understand the alcohol content of what you drink. See table. Drink low % drinks. Dilute high % drinks. Drink water between drinks to stay hydrated and decrease your total alcohol intake.

- Alcohol and violence go hand in hand. Stay away from individuals who become aggressive when drinking.

- Drinking lowers inhibitions and clouds judgment, resulting in violence, pregnancy, STDs.

- Never drink when you are pregnant or trying to become pregnant. It will cause fetal alcohol syndrome (birth defects).

- Do not mix medications with alcohol unless you have talked with the pharmacist and your doctor.

- Never mix drinking and hot tubs/saunas/etc. The massive vasodilation can be fatal.

• Alcohol is empty calories. One drink per day equates to 15 pounds per year of excess weight to deal with. Additionally, alcohol damages the liver, stomach and brain. Heavy drinking will cause cancer of the mouth, throat, breast and larynx.

• If you must drink, drink responsibly.

Alcohol Content

Beer 4-6% Malt Liquor 5-12% Wine 9-18%

Vodka, Gin, Whiskey, Rum, Brandy 35-80%

Grain Alcohol 85-95%

PROOF = (% of Alcohol) x 2

Example: 150 Proof Rum is 75% Alcohol

Hangover

Hangovers are the inevitable result of drinking. Despite hundreds of folk remedies, vitamins and quackery, no medically proven cure exists[6]. The cause is not entirely understood, but the severity of the hangover is dependant upon the drinker's weight and heredity, the amount and quality of spirit consumed and the stomach contents. Spirits contain the active ingredient ethanol (EtOH), along with toxic contaminants called congeners as well as the poison methanol. Further, alcohol is metabolized in the liver to formaldehyde (embalming fluid), and acetaldehyde, toxic poisons implicated in cirrhosis and alcoholism. EtOH is also a diuretic, causing dehydration and lowering blood glucose. All these factors contribute to the nasty syndrome known as a hangover.

Prevention and Preparation

The best prevention is not to drink at all. However, if you decide to drink, take a multivitamin, hydrate well and eat a normal meal. Healthy fats and carbs will slow digestion and EtOH absorption. Avoid alcohol with high congener levels. Congener levels are higher in cheap liquor, brandy, red wine and in darker liquors like rum, bourbon and scotch. Beer and white wine have a lower alcohol percentage and a moderate level of congeners. Distilled spirits like vodka and gin are cleaner. There are specialty vodkas now that are distilled four times and claim to be virtually congener free. Consider the type, quantity and quality of the alcohol you consume.

- Never drink more than one drink per hour.

- Stick to one drink or type of alcohol. Mixing causes trouble.

- Never play drinking games.

- Never drink unknown punch bowl concoctions.

- Alternate alcoholic drinks with glass of water with citrus wedge.

- Consider the mixer: Cola/energy drinks add up. Fruit juice is better.

- Let the designated driver monitor you.

Once Safely Home

- Hydrate and rest. Before bed, drink two full glasses of water or a sports drink, fruit juice, V8 or tomato juice.

- Take a multivitamin.

---

6 Pittler, M.H. *British Medical Journal*, Dec. 24-31, 2005; vol 331: pp 1515-1517.

- <u>Do not take analgesics!</u> Aspirin and NSAIDs can cause stomach ulcers/bleeding. Aetaminophen (Tylenol) when mixed with EtOH can cause liver failure.

The Morning After

- Avoid caffeine. It is another diuretic and stomach irritant.

- Forget "Hair of the Dog" which is an old English cure wherein the drinker attempts to treat his hangover by further drinking, a practice based on the medieval superstition that rabies could be prevented by placing the hair of the rabid dog into the wound. This treatment didn't work for rabies, nor will it work for a hangover. It only delays and worsens the inevitable.

Alcohol Poisoning

Excessive drinking, especially in short periods of time, can lead to alcohol poisoning. Binge drinking is linked to alcohol poisoning. As the alcohol blood level increases, it begins to depress normal body functions such as breathing, normal circulation and the gag reflex that protects our lungs and prevents choking. The most common cause of death is aspiration of the patient's own vomit and suffocation.

Symptoms

• Vomiting.

• Depressed or slow breathing, irregular pattern of breathing.

• Pale skin and in severe cases, bluish skin.

• Low body temperature.

• Seizure, unresponsiveness, unconsciousness.

Treatment

• If you suspect that someone has alcohol poisoning call 911 for assistance.

• If the person is breathing less than 8 times per minute, or is vomiting continuously, or unconscious and unresponsive: Call 911 immediately or the National Poison Control Center at 800-222-1222.

• Never leave a person with suspected alcohol poisoning alone.

Prevention

The best policy is drinking in moderation and only if over 21 years old. Drink beverages with low alcohol content. No binge drinking. No drinking games. Use a Breathalyzer to assess your blood alcohol content.

Drug Abuse

General Considerations

Drug abuse includes illegal drugs, prescription drugs, OTC drugs and alcohol.
Drug abuse has a crippling effect on the individual and on society. The costs are
staggering, estimated at $180 billion per year. The health risks are clear: Illegal drugs
are manufactured or processed in crude, unsanitary labs, then cut on the street with
contaminants (sugar, starch, baby powder, boric acid, strychnine) that can themselves
cause disease or death. IV drug use brings the added risks of HIV, AIDS and hepatitis.
But the full toll of drug use extends further: high risk behavior, financial costs,
felony convictions, increased street crime and the costs of addiction. Addiction is the
uncontrolled craving for a drug, often a physical dependence. Addiction occurs as
tolerance to the drug's effect develops, and higher doses are needed. The addict's life
revolves around obtaining the drug, and forestalling withdrawal. The physiological and
psychological effects of withdrawal are debilitating and life-threatening.

Cocaine

Cocaine is a powerfully addictive stimulant processed from the coca plant, originally
used as an anesthetic. Over 15% of Americans have used it. It can be snorted nasally,
injected directly into the veins, or smoked as 'crack' (named for the crackling sound
made when the rock is heated). Each route has unique levels of intensity and duration,
and repeated use can cause need for greater doses and addiction. Smoking and injecting
result in rapid onset and an intense but brief high. Crash is fast and hard. Higher and
higher doses are needed as tolerance develops. Health risks: heart disease, heart attack,
arrythmias, sudden death, lung disease, kidney disease, addiction.

Heroin

Heroin is a highly addictive derivative of morphine that has rapid onset and an intense
euphoric effect. It is a widely abused opiate, once urban but now spreading to a wider
demographic.

The white or brown powder or the black tar forms can be injected, snorted or smoked.
All forms and routes are addictive. Sensory rush is followed by long drowsy period,
depressed vital functions, often labored breathing resulting in death. Addiction is a
result of chronic changes in the brain pathways, and life revolves around getting the
drug at any cost. Health risks: bacterial sepsis, endocarditis, HIV, AIDS, hepatitis.

Oxycodone and Hydrocodone

Oxycodone is a pharmaceutical opiate with strength equal to morphine/heroin and a strong euphoric effect. The formulation Oxycontin® is a continuous release compound which jumpstarted painkiller abuse and took it to the top. Use is widespread across all age groups and social classes. Can be swallowed or crushed and snorted or injected. As addictive as heroin and more dangerous. Oxycodone is now the most common cause of lethal drug overdose in the US. Other health risks: liver damage from high acetaminophen load.

Marijuana

Marijuana, or pot, is the most commonly abused illegal drug in the US. It produces a euphoric state, altered perception and time distortion as well as paranoid and delusional thinking. The marijuana plant, *Cannabis Sativa*, has the active ingredients: THC or tetrahydrocannabinol and CBD or cannabidiol. There is long standing evidence of a link between THC and an increased risk of psychosis and schizophrenia. Recent studies suggest that CBD may counteract these changes in the brain. Unfortunately, the newly developed strains of 'skunk' super pot have very high concentrations of THC and minimal CDB. Furthermore, in some individuals these neurological changes are immediate and irreversible.

The history of marijuana in our country is fascinating, and driven more by emotion and politics rather than sound medical reasoning. While pot may have limited medical applications and a relatively low risk and addictive potential for most individuals, it has been shown to depress intellectual function for days after use and may result in prolonged suboptimal mental performance. The negative effects on scholastic and professional careers may be the true danger. Other health risks: onset of psychosis or schizophrenia, psychological and possible physical addiction, lowered testosterone levels.

MDMA (Ecstasy, X)

The greatest danger of MDMA is the misconception that this is a safe and benign "club drug". MDMA is a synthetic psychoactive derivative of methamphetamine with stimulant and psychedelic effects. It floods the brain with serotonin, causing damage to neural pathways. Studies show it may cause irreversible damage with just one dose. MDMA has an extremely high rate of dependence and risk of death from hyperthermia.

Methamphetamine (Meth, Speed, Crystal, Crank, Tweak)

Methamphetamine is a synthetic CNS stimulant with tremendous addictive potential. Many consider it the most serious and widespread drug threat in the US today. Broad demographic of college students, housewives, truckers, military personnel. Source is largely from Mexico but small local labs can cook meth simply from common OTC decongestants. Meth affects the dopamine brain pathway. Can be swallowed (Yaba is meth+caffeine pill), snorted, smoked or injected. It is a powerful stimulant causing euphoria and increasing energy, restlessness, heart rate and blood pressure. Secondary risks are aggressive and violent behavior, convulsions, stroke, heart attack, psychosis and advanced dental disease (meth mouth). Highly addictive, and the addiction is extremely difficult to treat.

Substance Abuse is a Serious Health Risk

The use of drugs, especially marijuana, has gone from a medical issue to a political one, and a growing deceptive trend is to characterize illegal drugs as lifestyle choices rather than crimes. Regardless of whether pot is a gateway drug, it is illegal. Possession can result in felony criminal charges with lifelong career, military service and credit rating implications. Lastly, it is wise to remember that alcohol is a drug, and that alcohol is far and away the most destructive, dangerous and prevalent substance ever abused. Alcohol is the only substance from which withdrawal can be fatal.

Drug Overdose

Drug overdose (OD) related fatalities in the US are increasing. OD and poisoning is the #2 accidental killer after motor vehicle accidents at a staggering cost of $10 billion per year. OD has many causes: too much or too pure drug, multiple drugs, drug interaction with alcohol or other drugs, intention ingestion of drug. Opioid painkillers (oxycodone) are the biggest killer by far, followed by cocaine, then heroin. In addition to the illegal drugs, OD occurs with prescription antidepressants and sedatives as well.

Symptoms and Signs of Drug Overdose

Diagnosing an OD is complicated, even for EMTs. There are too many unknowns: Type of drug? Quantity of drug? Combination of drugs? Alcohol? Injury? Existing medical conditions? There is no "typical OD"; e.g., opioids and cocaine have radically opposite effects. Symptoms and signs vary widely, especially in combination poisonings. However, OD presentation is usually a constellation of signs that something is very wrong with the patient:

Drowsy, unresponsive. Abnormal pupil size. Pupil nonreactive to light. Abnormal breathing patterns. Agitation, hallucination, irrational behavior. Abnormal body temperature. Abnormal heart rate and/or blood pressure. Abnormal clumsy or staggering gait. Skin cold/clammy or hot/flushed.

Dealing with an OD

A common and preventable cause of death in OD is vomiting and aspiration. This occurs because the gag reflex is lost and the patient is unable to keep vomit out of their lungs. Keeping them comfortable, calm and in the recovery position may save their life.

• First, assess the general situation to be sure you are safe and no dangers exist.

• Assess CAB: Circulation-Airway-Breathing.

• Call 911.

• Perform CPR if necessary.

• If patient is uninjured and breathing with pulse, place in the recovery position. This position allows secretions or vomit to drain freely from the mouth, and helps avoid aspiration. The position of the arms and legs prevents the patient from rolling back. Monitor closely.

- Dial <u>800.222.1222</u>. National Poison Control Center.

- Do not attempt to reason with or reprimand.

- Be careful. Drugs cause violent and unpredictable behavior. Protect yourself at all times.

- Monitor breathing and keep airway clear. Do not put fingers in mouth.

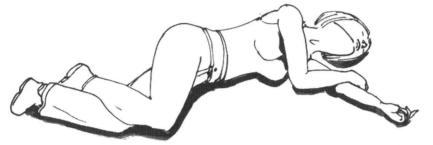

Drawing by Rama

The Recovery Position

Anabolic Steroids, DHEA, Growth Hormone and GHB

Anabolic steroids are a group of hormones related to testosterone that have the general effect of increasing muscle mass, bone density and virilization. The drugs are taken by pill, injection or skin patch. While they have limited medical use, illegal abuse by body builders and athletes to boost performance has serious and irreversible long term consequences.

Medical Alert: DHEA (Dehydroepiandrosterone)

DHEA is a hormone and precursor to testosterone and estrogen. The bizarre fact that it is classified as a "supplement" belies its potency; it is prohibited in Olympic competition and may soon be Rx only in the US. Although usually taken in the belief that increased DHEA levels will boost testosterone levels, the truth may be that estrogen levels are boosted even higher. DHEA may feminize males and virilize females, and may spur growth of hormone related cancers (breast, prostate, ovaries, testes). Side effects are similar to steroids. DHEA should never be taken without physician consultation.

Side Effects

Side effects in both sexes: violent and irrational behavior (steroid rage), acne, stunted growth (if taken before age 25), hypertension, heart attack, stroke, liver disease, liver cancer, baldness, depression, and:

♂: Erectile dysfunction, low sperm count, testicular atrophy, gynecomastia.

♀: Deep voice, rough skin, heavy facial and body hair, masculinization.

Some of these physical deformities can be grotesque and irreversible. There is evidence that steroid abuse leads to opioid abuse, making it a gateway drug. Added to these risks are the risks of impure, home lab contaminated drugs, and of IV drug usage if injecting the steroid: HIV and hepatitis.

Growth Hormone and GHB

Growth hormone stimulates development of muscle and bone. Normal production drops after adulthood. This drug and its precursors like GHB are abused by people believing that it will increase muscle mass or extend youth. In fact, the effects are just temporary; use must be continuous which causes irreversible deformities such as enlarged hands and feet and the facial bone thickening and the masculine features sometimes seen in female bodybuilders.

Side effects are similar to anabolic steroids: physical deformities, lactation in women, erectile dysfunction, diabetes, and hypertension. Growth hormone will energize cancer cells, accelerating the growth of an existing cancer. There is evidence that growth hormone may increase the risk of developing cancer as well.

Tattoos and Piercings

The popularity of body modification is at an all time high, chic and trendy. While many people love their choices and have no complications, many have regret. Unlike a bad haircut, tattoos are forever. Medical removal is extremely expensive, painful, protracted and always incomplete. Consider your choices wisely.

Tattoos

Tattoos are created by depositing pigment in the skin with needles. Professional tattoos place the color shallow, amateur tattoos (jailhouse tattoos) are usually deeper and therefore very difficult to remove. All tattoos should be considered permanent. The procedure breaks the defense of the skin, introduces foreign pigment to your immune system, and then leaves a large open sore as it heals, further exposing you to infection. Risks, other than pain and regret, include:

- Skin infection at tattoo site.

- Severe systemic allergic reaction to dye.

- Dermatitis/contact dermatitis at tattoo site.

- Ugly, raised, red (hypertrophic/keloid) scarring.

- Serious blood borne infectious disease: Hepatitis B, Hepatitis C, TB, tetanus, HIV, MRSA, 'flesh eating bacteria'. An outbreak of 44 cases of MRSA was traced to unlicensed tattoo artists; infection can occur if sterile procedure is not used. Sterile gloves, masks, autoclaved instruments and an antiseptic environment are essential.

- Secondary infection (transmission of disease either from the patient's open wound to a contact, or transmission of disease from an infected person into the patient's open wound) occurs, notably of MRSA.

Body Piercing

Piercing presents all the immediate risks of tattoos, and significantly greater long-term dangers, varying by site: ear cartilage (disfigurement), nipple (impaired breast feeding), mouth (poor speech, swallowed jewelry, gingivitis, broken teeth), navel (slow healing, scar, tears), genital (decreased sensation, torn condom with pregnancy or STD, impotence with male piercing).

Temporary Tattoos and Henna (Mehndi)

The FDA has seen adverse reactions to decal type temporary tattoos and henna. Henna is not approved for use on the skin. Avoid these tattoos; the safety of these products has not been fully determined.

Sexually Transmitted Diseases (STDs)

It is impossible to fully cover this crucial, life threatening topic in just a few pages. This brief overview is the basics only, and the reader should learn more at www.cdc.gov. It is essential that all sexually active people have a deep and complete understanding of STDs, pregnancy risks and safe sex practices. Regular testing is recommended, and should be discussed with your physician.

Mode of Transmission: V (vaginal sex) O (oral sex) A (anal sex)

Pelvic Inflammatory Disease (V)

PID is discussed first because it is common, serious, and difficult to diagnose and treat. PID is the infection of the female reproductive organs, usually by chlamydia or gonorrhea. The infection begins in the vagina, moves through the cervix and uterus, into the fallopian tubes and out into the abdominal cavity, causing inflammation, scarring and abscesses. Often early symptoms are mild or absent (silent), but the disease can develop into chronic severe abdominal pain, infertility, or ectopic pregnancies.

Chlamydia (VOA)

Chlamydia is a very common STD and virulent because it is silent and can destroy the reproductive organs of infected women resulting in infertility and an increased risk of HIV. Infection spreads untreated both in the individual and in the population because in 75% of women, there are no symptoms at all. In 40% of women, the disease progresses to PID. Yearly screening with a simple urine test is recommended, especially for sexually active females. Men may have urinary symptoms (discharge, discomfort). Although long term complications in men are rare, sterility can occur.

Gonorrhea (VOA)

Gonorrhea is a bacterial infection that is very common, and increasing in incidence. Transmission is VOA, symptoms may be present in males, but often are absent or mild in females and mistaken as yeast or bladder infections. Once established, the disease will cause PID, joint infections, and increase the risk of HIV. In pregnant women, the baby can be infected, blinded, or die. Diagnosis is by lab test, and all partners are treated with antibiotics.

Syphilis (VOA)

Syphilis is an important STD because it is increasing, can be silent and difficult to diagnose and if untreated can be fatal. It is more common in the South, in urban areas and in males. Transmission is VOA, and an open firm round painless chancre or sore may be present. A simple blood test can make the diagnosis. Early treatment is successful, but the late stages of the disease are progressive and untreatable.

Herpes Simplex Virus (VOA)

Herpes simplex viruses, HSV1 and HSV2, cause oral and genital herpes infections, infecting 25% of sexually active people, and in many there are no symptoms. There is no cure. The only defense is safe sex. Transmission is VOA, often asymptomatic, or with outbreaks of red blisters, the fluid of which is highly infectious. Herpes infection has been linked to increased risk of HIV even when the sores are healed, and can cause death or blindness of newborns. Infected individuals should abstain from sexual activity during outbreaks, and testing is crucial to diagnosis.

Hepatitis (VOA)

Hepatitis is a viral infection of the liver that is transmitted from person to person via the fecal-oral route or by blood and bodily fluids. There are three main types of hepatitis, A, B and C. Hepatitis A virus (HAV) is transmitted via the fecal-oral route and often obtained in areas of poor sanitation, unclean food establishment or in institutions. Hepatitis B (HBV) and C (HCV) are transmitted from person to person via the blood and bodily fluids. Tattoos have been implicated in the transmission of hepatitis C. The most common route of transmission is blood transfusions, IV drug use and sexual transmission. A vaccine is available for both HAV and HBV but not HCV. Most American children have been vaccinated with the hepatitis A and B vaccines.

Human Papilloma Virus (VOA)

Human papilloma virus (HPV) is the most common STD, infecting over half of sexually active adults. It is dangerous because often infection is asymptomatic and because it can cause genital warts, cervical cancer and cancers of the mouth, penis and anus. Venereal or genital warts, when they occur, can spread like wildfire into the vagina, cervix, penis, urethra and rectum. There are vaccines available to prevent the spread of HPV and vaccination is a crucial public health issue that is rapidly evolving. Consult your physician about whether vaccination is indicated for you. Treatment of HPV is difficult once contracted, and the infection may never be cured. Long-term follow-up may be required.

HIV and AIDS (VOA)

Human immunodeficiency virus or HIV, the virus that causes acquired immune deficiency syndrome or AIDS, is still infecting over fifty thousand people yearly in the US. Over half of transmissions are by people who do not know they are infected. Due to high risk sexual behavior, heterosexual infection is now more common than IV drug users, the infection rates for women are rising and half of all new infections are under the age of 25. While treatment options are improving, there is no cure. Individuals infected with HIV can be treated with medications to slow down the destruction of their immune system. AIDS is the late stage of the infection when the immune system is unable to fight disease and cancer. There are approximately 14,000 deaths from AIDS per year.

Prevention and Treatment of STDs

The best approach to all STDs is prevention by safe sex, or abstinence. You must realize that when you have sex with someone, you are having sex with every one of their past partners and their partners' partners, potentially hundreds of people. Many of these diseases have minimal or no symptoms. Regular screening and exams by a physician, total honesty in your sexual history and listing all partners for follow-up and treatment and compliance with the full regimen of antibiotics or treatment are absolutely essential. Many times patients stop taking drugs when the symptoms resolve, only to reinfect their partner and themselves.

Condoms

Condoms are like seatbelts. Use them every time, always, because you can never know or predict when you will need one to save your life. Remember that many STDs are asymptomatic or silent. One in four patients with herpes does not know that they have the disease, and will honestly, but incorrectly, tell you they are clean. Few healthy practices in life are as reliable, vital and inexpensive as wearing a condom. Use one every time.

Safer Sex

"Safer Sex" means to take precautions to minimize your risk of contracting an STD. Unprotected oral, vaginal or anal sex will expose you to the risk of contracting an STD. The use of condoms greatly reduces the risk of getting sexually transmitted disease. But only abstinence will protect you 100% from STDs and therefore is the only truly "Safe Sex" method.

- Consider abstinence.

- Consider a committed, monogamous relationship. Choose one partner and make sure you are their only partner. Get medical testing together to insure you are both STD free.

- Be selective in choosing partners. From the STD point of view, you are sleeping with everyone your partner has slept with.

- Drinking and taking drugs will alter your judgment and may lead to unsafe situations which you regret the next day and perhaps the rest of your life (HIV, pregnancy, hepatitis).

- Ask questions about your partner's sexual history and IV drug use. Do not be shy; your health and future is at risk. If your partner is not open with you, reassess having an intimate relationship.

- Take a look at your partner. Any sores or lesions, abstain from contact without a medical evaluation.

- Never have casual sex, hook ups or one night stands. You will not be their first.

- Use a latex condom <u>every</u> time you engage in oral, vaginal or anal sex. STDs occur from all types of sexual contact. Wear the condom before intimate contact for protection against STDs and pregnancy (pre-ejaculate can contain sperm).

- Only use <u>latex</u> condoms with reservoir tips and water based lubricant (Astroglide, K-Y Jelly).

- Use only water based lubricants; never use creams or lotions as they will cause the condom to break.

- Read the instructions for condom use, never open the package with your teeth, check expiration dates, never reuse a condom or use a damaged condom. If you do not follow instructions it won't protect you. Use it right. Go to <u>www.webMD.com</u> for links to tutorials and information.

- If a condom breaks, remove the condom and replace with a new one.

- Be careful when finished not to allow the condom to slip off. Remove and be careful not to spill contents.

• After disposing of a condom, wash your hands with soap and water.

• Spermicides kill sperm but are not considered effective against STDs. Use a condom.

• Be selective. Be prepared. Be smart.

Toxic Shock Syndrome

Toxic Shock Syndrome (TSS) is a rare condition caused by toxins invading the bloodstream from a staph or strep infection. TSS affects men and women and is of concern due to the rapid onset of severe symptoms, multiorgan system failure and a high mortality rate of 15%, sometimes within 48 hours.

Cause

TSS is associated with the use of tampons, the contraceptive sponge and the diaphragm/ cervical cap but is also seen in wound infections in both sexes. Not changing the tampon frequently, high/super absorbent tampons or contaminated wound dressings are implicated. Poor hygiene may play a role, as staph and strep bacteria are part of the normal skin flora.

Symptoms

The hallmark of TSS is sudden, severe flu-like symptoms: high fever, headache, sore throat, vomiting, diarrhea and a sunburn like rash. In wound infections, the site becomes red, swollen or painful. Low blood pressure, lightheadedness, bloodshot eyes, muscle aches may follow.

Treatment

Seek immediate medical care in TSS. Remove tampon or change wound dressing ASAP. Hospital treatment, support and IV antibiotics are critical to survival.

Prevention

TSS can be prevented with good hand washing hygiene prior to inserting tampons, avoiding tampons or alternating with pads and using low absorbency tampons. Read and follow carefully the instructions on tampons. Avoid continuous tampon usage during menstruation. Skin wounds should be cleaned and bandaged quickly after injury and bandages changed frequently.

Urinary Tract Infection (UTI)

Infections of the urethra (tube from bladder to outside) and bladder affect ten million Americans yearly, and 20% of women will have a UTI in their lifetime. Women are infected fifty times more often than men due to the short length of the female urethra and proximity of vaginal and anal bacterial flora, which cause almost 90% of UTIs. Rarely, herpes or yeast is implicated. Infection begins by the introduction of bacteria into the tip of the urethra, and then gradual ascending infection up the urethra to the bladder, and in severe cases, further up to the kidney itself.

Causes of UTI

Females – Poor hygiene, incorrect toilet habits such as wiping from back to front and seeding the urethra with fecal bacteria, intercourse, use of diaphragm with spermicide (the spermicide may inhibit/kill healthy vaginal bacteria and allow pathogens to flourish).

Males – Unprotected intercourse or anal intercourse, STDs (gonorrhea, chlamydia, herpes).

Symptoms and Signs

Females – Painful urination, urgent/frequent urination, cloudy/bloody urine.

Males – Yellow/green discharge, painful urination, urgent/frequent urination, cloudy/bloody urine.

Diagnosis and Treatment

Your physician will make the diagnosis based on your history, examination of a urine specimen, urine cultures and other tests. Treatment will vary depending on the cause of the UTI, but often requires antibiotics and teaching of effective prevention techniques. Women with more than three episodes of UTI yearly should have a thorough evaluation by their physician.

Prevention

• Prevention is key, especially in women. Recurrent UTIs can increase risk of permanent kidney damage.

• Drink cranberry juice (pure juice, no high fructose corn syrup) which acidifies the urine and is active against e.coli.

- Increase fluid intake so that urine output is "clear and copious". This washes out bacteria and prevents them from multiplying and ascending the urethra.

- Urinate immediately after sex.

- Practice proper hygiene: Wipe from front to back.

- Avoid diaphragms or condoms with spermicide.

- Avoid douching and hygiene products/sprays/deodorants as they tend to upset the natural vaginal flora.

- Change tampons or pads frequently.

Yeast Infections

Yeast infections are caused by the fungus *Candida Albicans* which exists in balance with harmless bacteria in both the vagina and the mouth. If the balance is upset, the fungus blooms causing oral thrush or vaginal yeast infections. This occurs from using antibiotics, oral inhalers (Advair), feminine hygiene sprays, douching or in immunosuppressed patients (diabetes, AIDS).

Symptoms

- Oral: raised white cheesy lesions, pain swallowing.
- Vaginal: thick white cheesy discharge, itching, pain.

Treatment

- A lab culture may be required.
- Oral: Your dentist may prescribe an oral antifungal drug.
- Vaginal: Your physician may recommend an OTC antifungal suppository or cream. Some infections require a prescription drug.
- If you have recurring infections, your doctor may recommend a blood test for diabetes or HIV or other evaluation.

Birth Control Warning

OTC antifungal suppositories and creams may
weaken condoms causing pregnancy or STDs.

Prevention

- To prevent oral thrush: Rinse mouth after using inhalers. Maintain good oral hygiene. Brush 3 times daily and floss. Do not use mouthwash as the alcohol or antiseptic upsets the normal balance of oral flora. Eat yogurt with probiotics when taking antibiotics.

- To prevent vaginal infections: Wash the vaginal area daily with unscented soap and water. Do not use scented toilet paper, deodorant sprays or deodorant tampons; the chemicals irritate the vaginal lining. Do not douche, which rinses away normal bacteria and secretions and can cause irritation or allergies. Unpleasant odors or discharge may be signs of infection. Normal vaginal discharge is minimal and either clear or white, but dries yellow on underwear. Wear cotton underwear which breathes better than synthetic fabrics, limit wearing pantyhose/spandex/tight pants, and change out of wet or damp workout clothes and swimsuits promptly.

• See your doctor or dentist for evaluation and treatment if you think you have an infection.

Oral Hygiene

Oral hygiene is of paramount importance to social success and health. Bad breath makes an unforgettable statement about your level of education and sophistication. Establishing and following a regular program of oral hygiene is a hallmark of good grooming. Bacteria thrive in the moist hot environment of the mouth, breaking down sugars into acid, causing tooth decay and bad breath. A thin sticky film of debris called plaque forms minutes after eating. Plaque has been linked to coronary artery disease and stroke. Over time, plaque calcifies into calculus, damaging gums and teeth. Here are the basics for healthy teeth and gums.

The Three Steps, in the Correct Order:
Brush, Floss, Irrigate

How to brush properly: See drawings.

• Brush your teeth with fluoride toothpaste after every meal for a minimum of two minutes.

• Fluoride strengthens enamel and fights cavities.

• Use only a <u>soft</u> toothbrush to prevent gum recession and replace every 3-4 months. Studies show that a brush with soft bristles and small head works best.

• Never share a toothbrush.

• Lastly, brush the tongue.

• A power toothbrush (Oral-B®, Sonicare®, Rotadent®) cleans your teeth far more thoroughly, removes stains better and stimulates gums. Highly recommended.

How to Brush

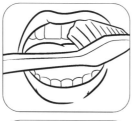

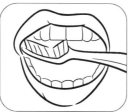

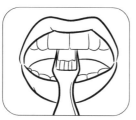

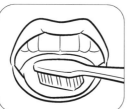

- Place the toothbrush at a 45-degree angle to the gums.

- Move the brush back and forth gently in short strokes.

- Brush the outer surfaces, the inside surfaces and the chewing surfaces of all teeth.

- To clean the inside surface of the front teeth, tilt the brush vertically and make several up-and-down strokes.

- Brush your tongue to remove bacteria and keep your breath fresh.

How to floss properly:

• You should floss every time you brush, but be sure to floss before bed.

• Pull out 14-18 inches of floss and wind around index fingers to guide.

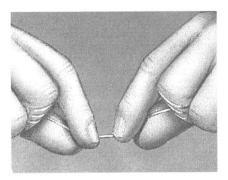

Image provided by Sunstar America, Inc.

• Gently guide in space between teeth, up/down, zigzag to clean.

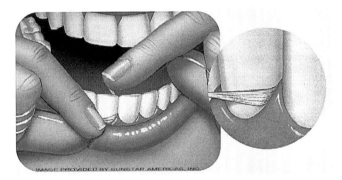

Image provided by Sunstar America, Inc.

• Do not hit or injure delicate gum tissue.

• Use clean section of floss for each tooth.

How to irrigate properly: Go to www.waterpik.com for information.

• Use clean fresh water only. No mouthwash or rinses.

• Irrigate gum line and between teeth for 3 seconds each.

• Waterpik® eliminates 99.9% of plaque in 3 seconds, and is excellent around orthodontia and dental work which may be difficult to floss manually.

• Clean the entire mouth.

Avoid sweets, eating between meals and visit your dentist twice a year for check-ups and cleanings.

Fractured or Avulsed Teeth

Dental trauma can be as simple as a small chip or as serious as fractured or avulsed teeth. Injury often occurs in sports, so when appropriate, a mouth guard should always be worn to protect your teeth and jaw. These are readily available at sports stores or can be custom made by your dentist.

Evaluation of Injury

Examine your mouth: Is there bleeding? Do your teeth fit together correctly? Are any teeth loose? Are any teeth chipped or broken? Does everything feel right? Do you have other injuries?

Treatment

If you have knocked out a tooth, you will need to see a dentist immediately to reposition and save the tooth. Call your dentist or local dental society (if you do not have a dentist, they will give you a referral) for emergency care. If you have other injuries, go to the ER.

Pick the tooth up by the crown not the root. Rinse it off in clean water if dirty. Place the tooth back in the socket if possible, or between your cheek and gum. The saliva will keep the tooth moist and healthy in its natural environment. If this is not possible then place the tooth in a cup of your saliva, milk or use Save-A-Tooth. Never scrub the tooth clean or transport the tooth dry. Try to get to the dentist within an hour as the success rate is higher if treated promptly. Your dentist will reimplant and stabilize the tooth.

Toothache

Dental pain or toothaches can be caused by a variety of problems such as dental cavities (caries), a cracked tooth, sinus problems, dental trauma or TMJ problems.

Causes and Treatment

• Dental caries or decay – This is the most common cause of dental pain. Bacteria break down sugar into acid that erodes dental enamel and exposes the sensitive pulp (nerve and blood supply) to bacterial toxins and environmental trauma (hot, cold, sweets). Treatment involves a visit to the dentist for the removal of decay and placement of a filling. In cases where the decay has gone deep into the tooth, a root canal (removal of pulp) or extraction may be required.

• Fractured or cracked tooth – Trauma may cause a crack or fracture in the tooth structure, exposing the pulp to the outside environment (heat, cold, bacteria). It can be minor trauma such as eating an un-popped kernel of popcorn or major trauma such as a motor vehicle accident. Biting on the tooth usually elicits pain specific to the tooth involved. Treatment would include a gold or porcelain crown to protect the tooth and prevent the crack from increasing. If the crack is deep, a root canal or extraction may be required.

• Periodontal disease – Pain can originate in the structures that surround the tooth: the gingiva (gum) and supporting bone. Failure to maintain good dental hygiene can result in inflammation of the gums, tooth loss, bone loss or infection. Regular cleaning by your dentist will remove the plaque that accumulates even with regular brushing.

• Other sources – Dental pain can come from other areas that "refer" the pain to your teeth. Common sources of pain are sinus infections, TMJ problems, ear infections and heart disease (a heart attack can refer pain to the jaw). Your dentist and physician will work together to determine the source of pain.

Wisdom Teeth

By young adulthood, the average adult has developed thirty-two teeth; sixteen teeth in the upper jaw and sixteen teeth in the lower jaw. However, the average mouth has room for only twenty-eight teeth. The wisdom teeth are the last four molars to erupt, and in early humans were meant to replace teeth lost to wear or disease. Today, modern dental care and antibiotics insure that teeth are rarely lost, our diet is softer and the human jaw is slightly smaller. Orthodontic treatment creates a full dental arch and does not leave room for additional teeth to erupt. As a result of all these factors, often there is no room for the wisdom teeth to erupt. They become impacted below the surface of the gums or grow at odd angles, causing complications. Impacted wisdom teeth create problems such as infections, decay, gum disease, orthodontic crowding, and cysts or tumors of the jaws.

Symptoms

Impacted wisdom teeth can be asymptomatic, however if complications occur, you may experience the following symptoms:

• Dental or jaw pain

• Swelling around the wisdom tooth with discharge

• Inflamed gums

• Facial or jaw swelling

• Limited jaw opening

• Unpleasant taste and odor

• Headache

• Fever

Treatment

If you have any symptoms, you should immediately visit or call your dentist for a referral to an oral surgeon for evaluation. Your oral surgeon will usually take an x-ray, examine the area of concern, prescribe antibiotics, give home care instructions and schedule the removal of wisdom teeth under IV anesthesia. If impacted wisdom teeth are asymptomatic, removal is also indicated in most cases. By removing asymptomatic impacted wisdom teeth at a younger age, potential future problems (infections, cysts, tumors) are eliminated and the surgical risks of the procedure are significantly reduced.

Temporomandibular Joint (TMJ) and Disorder (TMD)

The TMJ is a dual joint complex that uses a unique gliding motion to open, close, talk, bite and yawn. Within the TMJ a cushioning disc glides back and forth as the jaw opens and closes. Malfunction or inflammation of the joint, disc or muscles results in facial/ jaw pain, often called Temporomandibular Disorder.

Causes

When the TMJ or supporting muscles are traumatized, the joint can become temporarily or permanently injured. Joint injury or muscle fatigue may be caused by low-grade chronic trauma (clenching or grinding the teeth) or more violent, acute trauma (automobile accident or assault). The social and academic pressures of college may cause an increase in stress-related clenching and grinding resulting in TMD. Injuries may cause disc displacement, disc erosion, arthritic bony changes or muscle inflammation. All can result in various degrees of pain and dysfunction.

Symptoms

Facial pain can come from numerous sources such as a toothache, sinus infection, gum disease or TMD. Temporomandibular disorders may present as pain, popping or clicking in the TMJ, limited opening, muscle soreness, malocclusion (misaligned bite), pain with chewing, waking up at night with pain, ear pain and joint swelling. In severe cases, the TMJ may lock closed or open. Consult your dentist for evaluation of facial pain.

Treatment

Temporomandibular disorders are best treated with conservative and reversible non-surgical therapies. These include a soft diet, cold compresses, physical therapy, joint rest, orthodontics or adjustment of your bite. Initially, pain medications should be limited to OTC NSAIDs (Advil, Aleve). Your dentist or physician may prescribe muscle relaxants or antidepressants to relieve persistent symptoms. If muscles are the source of pain, referral to a physical therapist is often recommended. When clenching is the causative factor, a custom acrylic splint or night guard is fabricated by your dentist. In rare cases, surgical treatment is required.

Bites, Stings and Venom

Most animals have defense mechanisms, and many include biting, clawing or stinging. Some have venom and in others it is the bacteria in saliva that is harmful. In fact, with human bites and cat bites, it is the secondary bacterial infection that is the most virulent.

Animal Bites – Dogs, cats, wild animals. If possible, quarantine the animal and notify police. Dog bites involve a significant crush component; cat bites are puncture wounds that can become deep tissue infections. Seek medical attention immediately.

Human Bites – Common, with the main danger being bacterial infection from saliva. A "fight bite" occurs when the fist strikes the mouth, and often results in a tendon laceration and rapid, serious hand infections. All human bites should be immediately seen by a physician and antibiotics given as needed.

Snake Bites – Pit vipers (rattlesnakes, copperheads, cottonmouths) cause most venomous snake bites in the US. Surprisingly, up to half of bites may be "dry", with no venom injected, so do not panic. The victim should be taken immediately to the ER. If possible, photograph or describe the snake as the proper antivenin must be given. Remove any constricting clothing, jewelry, etc. from the limb, transport with limb below level of heart. Do not attempt any X cutting of the area of the bite, sucking of venom, tourniquet or other cure, as they are ineffective and may be harmful. With prompt care and the proper antivenin, the prognosis is excellent.

Spider Bites – While nearly all spiders are venomous, few are large or powerful enough to break human skin. The female black widow with a red hourglass mark on her abdomen, and the brown recluse with a violin shape on its body and telltale bull's-eye bite mark, are the two spiders of concern to humans. The immediate symptom of a spider bite is pain and the best treatment is an ice cube to the site. Medical treatment may be required, but these bites are rarely fatal.

Flying Insects – Bees, wasps, hornets. Humans can survive ten stings per pound of body weight, meaning the average male can survive over a thousand stings. These beneficial insects rarely sting unless protecting the queen or the hive, or provoked. If stung, first get far away from the insects. Treatment requires that the stinger be removed immediately, using fingers or scraping with a credit card. Use an ice cube for pain, and a topical antihistamine and corticosteroid cream. Medical treatment is rarely needed, except in cases of allergy or anaphylactic reaction, which can be fatal.

Scorpion Stings – The scorpion is a predator, and uses its venomous sting to immobilize and kill its prey. Most American scorpions have a mild sting; the exception is the bark scorpion found in the desert southwest whose toxin is much stronger. Treatment is an ice cube for pain, and a topical antihistamine and corticosteroid cream. Medical treatment may be necessary for the bark scorpion sting.

Eye Injuries

There are 2.5 million eye injuries yearly in the US, and almost half occur in the home. The July 4th weekend is notorious for a high incidence of eye injuries.

Causes of Injuries

- Microwave – Steam or hot liquids, popcorn bag steam, hyperheated eggs.
- Chemicals – Splash of acid, alkali, pool and household chemicals.
- UV light – Sunlight and tanning salons.
- Wind, dust, snow – Outdoor activities and particulate matter into eye.
- Machines, hammers, impact tools – High speed metal or other fragments.
- Bungee – Unexpected breaking or release.
- Lacerations – Direct trauma to eyelids and/or eye.

Treatment

Treatment can be very difficult due to the intense, blinding pain involved in many eye injuries as well as the victim's loss of vision. The best strategy is prevention.

- Never attempt removal of a high velocity metal fragment, or any sharp fragment, from the eye. Go immeidatly to the ER.
- Wash your hands to be sure not to introduce further dirt or bacteria into the eye.
- Never wipe the eye with a cotton swab, your finger or anything else. This can only introduce bacteria and drive a foreign body or sharp fragment deeper into the eye tissue, possibly causing permanent damage or blindness.
- Wash the eye immediately and thoroughly, especially in chemical splashes. Saline eye wash is preferable, however clean tap water is perfectly good and far more available. Rinse for a minimum of twenty minutes. Use a water fountain, a kitchen faucet, the shower, a glass or the garden hose (on low pressure).
- If the rinse fails to remove the irritant, open the eye wide and in a well lit area, examine the eye. Look up, down, right, left. Localizing the foreign body may make it easier to wash it out. Try to keep eyelid open; excessive blinking or closing the eyelid on an injury can actually increase the damage.

Prevention

Imagine your life without vision. The challenges would be immense. Buy and use quality eye protection. Keep a pair of safety glasses that comply with the ANSI standards handy and use them. www.labsafety.com. Always wear sunglasses to protect from UV and glare. Use common sense in July 4th celebrations and exercise caution with fireworks, explosives and sparklers.

Eye Infections

Stye and Chalazion

A stye (hordeolum) is an infection of an oil gland in the eyelid, often caused by staph bacteria. The duct of the gland becomes plugged, and swelling, infection and tenderness follow. Chalazions are very similar to styes, but tend to be larger, slow growing but not painful because they are not infections. They are caused by blockage of the oil duct, with resultant swelling and rupture of the gland into surrounding eyelid tissue. The two conditions can be difficult to differentiate, however their causes and treatment are similar and they are usually benign and resolve without treatment. Both are caused by poor facial and eyelid hygiene, rubbing your eyes with dirty hands, excessive makeup and old or infected makeup and makeup tools, brushes and curlers. Makeup can become colonized with bacteria, and has a maximum life of six months.

Symptoms and Signs

• Redness

• Swelling or lump

• Pain

• Discharge when they drain.

Treatment

• Be patient. Most will resolve with home treatment.

• Clean gently with baby shampoo.

• Warm, wet compresses 4-6 times daily.

• Do not squeeze or attempt to "pop". Allow them to drain on their own.

• No makeup or contact lenses until healed.

• If no improvement with home treatment, seek medical attention.

Prevention

• Wash hands before touching your eyes.

• Never share makeup, makeup tools or brushes.

• Discard makeup, especially mascara and eyelid brushes, after six months.

• Keep your eyelashes and eyelids clean by washing your face every morning and evening. Baby shampoo works well for cleansing eyelids and eyelashes.

Conjunctivitis (Pink Eye)

Conjunctivitis is an inflammation of the conjunctiva (the covering of the eye and eyelids). It is caused by a bacterial or viral infection and on occasion by allergies. The infectious forms are extremely contagious and transmitted by contact with finger, washcloth or towel.

Symptoms and Signs

- Conjunctiva of eye is red or pink.
- Eye feels gritty when blinking.
- Discharge may be present and overnight becomes crusty.
- Bacterial infections produce a thick, yellow discharge.
- Viral infections may cause sore throat and swollen lymph nodes.
- Allergic conjunctivitis causes a clear discharge.

Treatment

- Your doctor may take a sample for laboratory analysis.
- Bacterial conjunctivitis is treated by gently rinsing with warm water and prescription antibiotic eye drops. Resolves in one week.
- Viral conjunctivitis resolves in 7 to 10 days with washing only.
- Allergic conjunctivitis should be treated by your doctor with eye drops and evaluation of possible allergens.

Prevention

- Wash your hands frequently with soap and water.
- Use only your own towels and washcloths. If you have an infection, change them daily.
- Always wash your towels, sheets and pillowcases in hot water.
- See your physician for a thorough evaluation if you develop symptoms.

Acne

Acne is caused by clogging of pores by dirt, body oil called sebum, and the bacteria *Propionibacterium acnes*. Sebum is produced more as hormones increase, causing young adult acne. There are four types of acne:

- Whitehead – sebum blocks and seals the pore.

- Blackhead – sebum blocks the pore then oxidizes to black.

- Pimple – bacteria infect a blocked pore causing redness and inflammation.

- Cyst – inflammation is severe and pus accumulates.

Basics of Skin Care for Acne

Never pick, squeeze or pop acne. This prolongs healing and may cause scarring.

Avoid astringents, alcohol or exfoliants. These irritate and dry skin, causing breakouts. Only benzoyl peroxide or salicylic acid will help clear your acne. Other products can make it worse.

Do not touch your face. Introducing bacteria from your hands to your face causes acne.

Shaving – Moisten hair with warm water (shave after showering). Shave lightly; never shave or cut acne. Try an electric razor to assess which gives you better results.

OTC treatments – Benzoyl peroxide reduces the bacterial count on your skin and removes dead skin. Salicylic acid helps prevent acne by unclogging pores. Seek a dermatologist's help if you have severe acne.

How to Wash Your Face

Wash your face twice daily, in the morning and evening. If you perspire heavily, wash your face immediately afterward. Hats, helmets and headbands will make acne worse. Hair products, make-up and skin products should be oil-free.

- Use a non-abrasive cleanser with no alcohol.

- Use your fingertips. Do not use a washcloth, sponge or puff as they irritate skin.

- Rinse with lukewarm water.

- Shampoo every day and if you use a conditioner, use it before washing your face. Conditioners can cause acne, especially back acne.

- Apply OTC products (benzoyl peroxide or salicylic acid) 5-15 minutes after washing your face. Wet skin is too absorbent and these products will cause irritation. Apply makeup after acne products. Go to www.aad.org for more information.

Dandruff

Dandruff is caused by dead flakes of skin that develop on the scalp. The most common causes of dandruff are seborrheic dermatitis and psoriasis. Hair is not affected.

Treatment

- Use an over the counter shampoo daily with one or more of these ingredients: tar, selenium, sulfur, salicylic acid, zinc or ketoconazole.

- Lather twice each time you shampoo. First time for one minute and the second time for 5 minutes.

- If your dandruff persists, see a dermatologist for prescription shampoo or corticosteroid lotion.

Athlete's Foot, Ringworm and Jock Itch

Both athlete's foot and jock itch are caused by a fungus called *Tinea*. Tinea infects the skin, hair or nails and grows in a circular, ring like fashion. The edge of the ring is red and scaly, making it look like a worm under the skin, thus it is sometimes called ringworm. It occurs from contact with fungus in showers, bathrooms, dorm rooms, locker rooms and even from family pets.

Symptoms

- Dry skin that is red, flaky and itchy.
- Moist skin is white and soggy.
- Athlete's foot may involve the nails.
- Jock itch appears in the upper inner thigh area.
- Your doctor can take a sample for microscopic evaluation to confirm the presence of a fungus and confirmation of the clinical diagnosis.

Treatment

- OTC antifungal cream (Tinactin).
- Apply cream twice per day for 2 to 4 weeks.
- Dry skin after showering.
- Throw out old shoes that the fungus has contaminated and colonized.
- If the OTC antifungal creams fail to eliminate the infection, your doctor may prescribe a stronger cream or an oral anti-fungal medication.

Prevention

- Change socks and underwear every day.
- In hot weather, avoid thick clothing and try to wear sandals or shoes that are breathable.
- Air out your shoes when not wearing them.
- Use sandals in locker rooms or dorm bathrooms. Never walk barefoot!
- Never share towels, bathmats or nail clippers.
- Check your pets for fur loss and take to veterinarian for treatment.
- Use anti-fungal cream if someone in the house or dorm close to you has athlete's foot to prevent the fungus from infecting you.

Sleep Deprivation

Seventy million Americans suffer from sleep deprivation, a largely undiagnosed disease more harmful than smoking, resulting in poor performance in school, work and play. Adults need 7-9 hours of good sleep to restore mind and body. Too little, poor quality, or even too much sleep reduces alertness, memory, mental acuity, even life expectancy. Studies attribute sleep disorders as causing over 100,000 auto accidents yearly. The risk increases for job injury, heart attack, stroke, obesity, depression and birth defects. Luckily, it is preventable.

Develop a Pre-sleep Ritual:

• Establish a routine and stay on it, even on the weekends – Daily exercise helps sleep. Stop eating/drinking 2 hours before bedtime, wind down physical and mental activity, and prepare yourself to sleep.

• No caffeine, tea, cola, or alcohol (impairs dreaming).

• No smoking, tobacco, snuff.

The Bedroom Environment

Think cave: dark, quiet and cool.

• The bedroom should be very dark, even faint light disrupts sleep.

• Quiet is essential. If necessary and safe, use soft earplugs.

• The bedroom is for sleep or intimacy. TV/laptops etc. can disrupt sleep.

• Bedroom should be cool; studies show 68° is ideal.

• Put pets in another room. Animals (and their hair, dander and mites) cause allergies/dermatitis. They move and disrupt your sleep.

• Bedding – get a good quality mattress that you love, you spend a third of your life on it. Follow manual re: flip/spin/when to replace. Technology has changed, but mattresses have a lifespan. Use allergen barrier mattress pad and high quality sheets, and wash them weekly in hot water.

• Pillows – use foam/synthetic pillows. They are less allergenic and can be washed easily. Pillows are a major cause of neck and back pain, and incorrect use is common. Evaluate how you sleep (back/belly/side) for the best choice of pillow.

Medications – Never use Rx sleep medications unless directed by a physician. There are serious risks. OTC medications have risks of daytime drowsiness. Melatonin has not been proven to be an effective therapy, and may actually throw off normal circadian rhythms.

Bed Bugs

Bed bug infestation has plagued mankind forever. These small, white or brown parasites feast on human blood, usually living in bedding or in furniture. They are found in hotel rooms, theaters, airplane seats, even retail stores. Nearly wiped out last century, they are returning with a vengeance due to the banning of effective pesticides.

Like mosquitoes, they suck blood painlessly. The bites become red, raised and itch. Disease transmission risk is low but recent studies have shown that methicillin resistant staphylococcus aureus (MRSA) can be carried and spread by bed bugs. Additionally, the bites can become infected and are aggravating. Diagnosis can be difficult as flea, mosquito, chigger bites are very similar in appearance.

Prevention

The best approach is prevention. Bed bugs hitchhike into your home on your luggage and clothes. Travel brings you in contact with them.

- Keep your luggage off the floor in hotel rooms.
- Immediately inspect the mattress/pad/sheets/walls for brown spots/streaks (feces).
- When you return home, keep the luggage in the garage, and vacuum inside and out to remove any hitchhiking bed bugs.
- Launder clothes in hot water or dry clean.
- Don't buy used mattresses or furniture.

Treatment

Once infestation has occurred, elimination of the elusive pests is difficult and expensive. Do not attempt to do this yourself. Hire a licensed professional. Even then, it may take multiple treatments.

Lyme Disease

Lyme disease is a bacterial infection caused by *Borrelia Burgdorferi* transmitted by deer ticks, and first identified in 1975 in Lyme, Connecticut. Deer ticks live in grassy and heavily wooded areas. Wood ticks and dog ticks do not carry Lyme disease, but can carry other diseases. Rural housing developments and a rise in the deer population has doubled the incidence of Lyme disease.

Symptoms

- A telltale bull's eye circular rash occurs in 70% of patients.

- Fever, chills, swollen lymph nodes, headaches and fatigue.

- Stiff neck, muscle aches, joint pain.

- Advanced cases develop arthritis, nerve and heart problems.

Diagnosis and Treatment

- Remove and freeze the tick for lab examination.

- Seek medical care if you suspect Lyme disease. Diagnosis and treatment is easier in the early stages of the disease. If you have a bull's eye rash, take a picture. Your doctor may also take blood tests to measure antibodies.

- Treatment of Lyme disease is with antibiotics. Most patients are cured in a few weeks if treated immediately. Patients in the later stages of the disease require additional antibiotics and the success rate is not as high. Get early treatment.

Prevention

- Avoid grassy, heavily wooded areas. Stay on the trails. Keep to the center of the path and keep your body off the ground. Wear light colored long pants, shirts and socks so ticks are visible. Tuck cuffs and apply DEET to clothing to prevent ticks getting under clothes.

- Be especially careful during summer when ticks are most active.

- The CDC recommends DEET (20-30%) on exposed skin. 20% DEET provides about 4 hours of protection; reapply every 4 hours.

- Wear tick resistant Permethrin treated clothing (Insect Shield®) or put DEET or Permethrin on clothing. Permethrin kills ticks on contact. Permethrin treated clothes can be purchased or you can buy Permethrin solution and treat your clothes. Permethrin should not be applied to skin.

• After an outing, check entire body, especially areas that get moist: underarms, backs of knees, groin, navel, buttocks, neck, ears. Shower and shampoo with warm water ASAP.

How to Remove a Tick

Ticks do not just suck blood like a mosquito; they bury their mouth parts under the skin. Proper technique must be used in removal, or the head remains embedded causing infection, irritation and inflammation.

<u>The tick must be removed alive</u>.

<u>Do Not: Burn, heat or use alcohol or chemicals on the tick</u>.

Proper Technique

Using blunt delicate tweezers and latex gloves, gently grasp as close to the head as possible. Do not squeeze or crush the body. This will spill bacteria. Gently pull outward. Do not twist or jerk. Pull enough to tent up the skin and gradually ease out the tick's head. Pull for 3-4 minutes as it lets go and backs out. Check to see you got it all. Put in plastic bag and freeze it. If you get sick, take it for analysis. Wash bite area thoroughly with soap and alcohol.

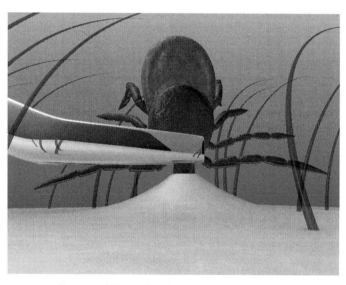

Courtesy of Centers for Disease Control www.cdc.gov

Dust Mites

Dust mites are microscopic vermin. They love humans, pets, warmth, humidity and dead human skin cells. They thrive in mattresses, pillows, bedding, upholstery and carpeting. While they don't bite or transmit disease, they are the most common cause of household allergies, asthma, skin problems and sleep disorders due to irritation from their body parts and feces.

Prevention and Treatment

Eliminating favorable environments for dust mites will control the allergen load.

- Avoid dust collectors (fabric upholstery, drapes, carpet, down comforters, etc.). Hard flooring is preferable to carpeting.

- Vacuum with HEPA filter frequently. HEPA filter traps allergens. Use N95 mask (blocks 95% of small particles) while cleaning.

- Use encasements on box spring, mattress, pillowcases, and duvet. These act as impenetrable barriers for dust mites, bedbugs, mold and other allergens.

- Buy new mattresses every 5-10 years. Half the weight of a 10 year old mattress is dust mites and dust mite feces.

- Steam clean carpets every spring.

- Keep bedrooms especially clean. Keep pets out and make their sleeping area as far away as possible. Vacuum mattress often, and wash all bedding in hot water weekly, using hot dryer.

- Air Filters – www.EPA.gov recommends HEPA filters. Do not use ozone air filters. They are ineffective and may be hazardous to your health. Use only high efficiency furnace filters with MERV rating >12 to remove airborne allergens.

- Travel: Take a pillow encasement on trips for hotel rooms. Shower and launder clothes upon return.

NUTRITION

"Man is what he eats."

Ludwig Feuerbach 1804-1872

Nutrition 101

You are what you eat. You are constantly changing, growing, healing, repairing and aging, tearing down and rebuilding, as long as you live. The sole source of essential building blocks for rejuvenation is the food you eat, your diet. Unfortunately our high fat, highly processed American diet is both deficient and a major contributing factor for obesity. Obesity is epidemic in the US, with 70% of Americans overweight. Obesity results in diabetes, heart disease, vascular disease, breast cancer, colon cancer, arthritis, hypertension, shortened lifespan, poor quality of life, diminished self image and more. The effects of a poor diet are cumulative, and difficult to reverse. The first step to a healthy body is a healthy diet.

The Basics of Nutrition: Carbohydrate, Protein and Fat

- Carbohydrate – Carbs are the basic fuel of the body and come in the form of sugars, starches and complex carbohydrates. Your body breaks them down to glucose to use as fuel or to store as glycogen. Excess becomes fat.

- Fat – Fatty acids, lipids and cholesterol are vital to body function, brain, skin, hormones.

- Protein – The structure and function of the body depends on protein: muscle, skin, bone, enzymes and hormones. Protein is long chains of 20 amino acids (aa), 13 that our body can make, and 9 (essential aa) we must obtain in our daily diet.

- Vitamins – 13 vitamins are needed in cellular reactions and metabolism. They cannot be made by the body, and therefore dietary intake is needed, but too much can be toxic.

- Phytochemicals (*phyto* means plant in Greek) – Compounds found in fruits, vegetables, beans, nuts and grains. Unlike vitamins, they are not essential for human life but have been shown to have significant health benefits, including anti-aging and protection against cancer and heart disease.

- Minerals – Calcium for bones, teeth. Iron (especially females) for blood. Electrolytes. Trace elements. Zinc for wound healing. All are critical for health and normal metabolic function.

- Water – Hydration keeps cellular processes working, the blood from sludging and maintains a good oxygen supply to the organs. Adequate hydration is essential to flush toxins through the kidneys. Use thirst and urine output and color (clear and copious) to gauge hydration.

- Dietary Fiber – Indigestible carbohydrate of plant origin that promotes health in many ways and is severely lacking in our highly processed Western diet.

Carb/Fat/Protein Ratio – There is much made of the proper ratio of carbohydrate to fat to protein in your diet. The reality is that there is no magic formula; and if there was, it would be nearly impossible to implement on a daily basis. Your body does not care what form energy comes in; it will use anything you eat. The key is simple: Do not overeat. Excess calories, whether carb, fat or protein, will become fat. Avoid supersizing.

Heart Healthy Diets – There is little question that a high fat diet contributes to heart disease; furthermore, recent studies indicate that certain low fat diets can slow and perhaps even reverse cardiovascular disease. Research shows that arterial plaque can actually disappear when patients follow a low fat, vegetarian diet and exercise. www.WebMD.com has excellent reviews of several low fat and heart healthy diets.

Carbohydrates

Carbohydrates are our primary, most efficient energy source, and the building blocks of DNA and RNA. Carbs have many names: sugars, starches and fiber. They exist in many forms ranging from simple sugars like glucose and fructose to complex carbohydrates, long chains of thousands of sugars linked together, like glycogen. They have been the mainstay of our diet since the dawn of time. The absorption, metabolism and storage of carbs are critical to optimal mental performance and health because the human brain can only use glucose as fuel; low blood glucose levels impair brain function.

Carbohydrate Metabolism

- Complex carbs like fruits and starches must be broken down by gastric enzymes to be absorbed; this process leads to a slow, gradual rise in blood glucose. Insulin moves the glucose into cells for fuel and stores any excess as glycogen in the liver and muscle. Later, glycogen releases glucose molecules for fuel and to maintain stable blood glucose levels.

- Simple sugars, like glucose and fructose, are easily absorbed and elevate blood sugar too quickly, causing a sharp spike of insulin. The overload of insulin signals the body to store the glucose as fat, not glycogen. This storage of sugar as fat is a major cause of the obesity epidemic.

- Glycemic Index (GI) – Developed by DJ Jenkins, MD from the University of Toronto as a method for controlling diabetes, the GI is a scientifically determined measure of how quickly a specific food elevates blood glucose. The GI of pure glucose is 100, and foods are ranked HIGH>70, MED 56-69, LOW <55.

- Glycemic Load (GL) – Developed at Harvard University, GL measures both the GI and the load of carb in a normal serving of a food, and is a more useful tool. LOW <10, MED 11-19, HIGH > 20. But even the GL is not the entire answer; fiber, fat and acid content as well as mixing of different types of foods in a meal all affect the absorption of glucose.

Evidence has shown that high GI/GL foods like a donut for breakfast cause rapid peaks in blood glucose, followed by overproduction of insulin and lipids. The net effect is an increased risk of obesity. A diet using low GI/GL foods has significant advantages in weight control and may actually be more important in managing cholesterol than fat intake.

- LOW GL – Bran cereals, whole grain/wheat/rye bread, fruits, peas, beans, black beans, carrots, corn, edamame, popcorn, lentils, legumes, beets, peanuts, low-fat ice cream, milk, yogurt, soy milk.

- MED GL – Fruit juices, wild rice, brown rice, sweet potato, cereals, soft drinks, breakfast bars, cookies, crackers, chips.
- HIGH GL – White rice, pasta, fries, couscous, potatoes, muffins, pastries, candy, raisins, dates, energy bars.

It is important to use GL to guide nutritional choices. Be aware that portion sizes often used in charts are petite, and don't forget to add other components like salad dressings, croutons, etc. when calculating calories for your meal. Remember, 2000 calories of salad is still 2000 calories.

Dietary Fiber

Fiber, bulk or roughage consists of soluble and insoluble carbs that can't be digested or absorbed but are vital to health. Fiber gives a feeling of fullness, lowers BP, slows absorption of sugars and holds water. Soluble fiber lowers blood cholesterol by binding with bile and dietary cholesterol. Insoluble fiber cleanses the gut.

- The average American gets less than half of the daily recommended intake of fiber, a deficiency that contributes to our obesity.
- Suggested Intake – ♀25gm/day, ♂35gm/day.
- Soluble Fiber – Oatmeal, apples, citrus, beans, peas, lentils, bran, potatoes, sweet potatoes.
- Insoluble Fiber – Whole grains, bran cereals, cabbage, broccoli, cauliflower, beets.
- Supplements – Many forms: pills, powders, candy, liquids. Consult your physician and experiment to find the best one for you.

Incorporating fiber into a healthy diet aids in weight management, and lowers risk of diabetes, heart disease and cancer.

Fat

The American high-fat diet has been implicated in increasing the risk of obesity, heart disease, colon, prostate and breast cancer, autoimmune disease, stroke, Alzheimer's, depression, hypertension, impotence and diabetes. But fat is not all bad. Fat is the most concentrated form of energy, and is essential for cell membrane turnover, skin, hormones and Vitamin A, D, E and K function. It is the fat in a meal that gives the feeling of fullness and satiety. And certain fats may actually reverse heart disease.

The Basics of Fat

- Cholesterol – Long vilified, cholesterol is essential for membrane function, hormone production and digestion. Only 20% of blood cholesterol is from our diet; 80% is made in our liver as two compounds: Low Density Lipoproteins (LDL or bad cholesterol) and High Density Lipoproteins (HDL or good cholesterol). Recent studies implicate LDL in plaque buildup in blood vessels, causing heart attacks, stroke, vascular disease, and increased risk of breast and colon cancer. High levels of HDL have a protective effect, and actually lower the levels of LDL. The LDL/HDL balance is critical to good health and while it is partially genetic, it can be improved by diet and exercise.

- Saturated Fat – Bad fat. Found in red meat, poultry skin, lard, butter, whole dairy, palm oil and coconut oil. Saturated fat will increase LDL and disease risk. Avoid this fat like the plague.

- Unsaturated Fat – Healthy fat. Found in the good vegetable oils, nuts, seeds, peanuts and avocado. Canola and olive oil are known to lower LDL, prevent and maybe even reverse heart disease and dissolve plaque.

- Trans Fat – The worst fat of all. A small amount of trans fat exists in nature, but the vast majority is synthetic. Used to chemically solidify liquid oils into hard margarine and other processed foods, it is toxic. The American Heart Association says <2gms/d. Avoid trans fat in any form or amount.

- Triglycerides – The main form of fat in the body, triglycerides are used as fuel or transported in the blood to fat cells for storage. Triglycerides are formed from fatty meals, from the excess sugar when blood glucose is elevated after a large meal, or when sweet drinks or alcohol is ingested. High levels of triglycerides result in deposition of body fat and may increase the risk of heart disease. Alcohol sharply increases blood triglycerides, and a low fat diet and omega 3 fatty acids act to lower blood triglycerides.

• Essential Fatty Acids – EFAs cannot be synthesized by the body, and must be part of our diet. Two types of EFA exist in a delicate balance that determines our health: omega 3 vs. omega 6. Unfortunately, our diet has too much omega 6 and not enough omega 3. Increased intake of natural omega 3, found in oily fish like salmon and in canola oil and flaxseed oil, has profound, whole body health benefits.

Tropical Oils: The Bad Vegetable Oils

American Heart Association recommends avoiding the three tropical oils because they have very high levels of heart clogging saturated fat: coconut oil (92%), palm kernel oil (82%), palm oil (50%). Often labeled as healthy vegetable oils, they are hidden in a many foods: baked goods, cookies, cakes, pastries, peanut/hazelnut/almond butter, snack foods, granola, protein and energy bars. Check the ingredient list on all foods.

The Good Fats

Dietary fat is unavoidable, and necessary. Just as saturated fat is harmful to health, unsaturated fats and omega fatty acids can be beneficial to health. When cooking, one must remember that all oils are pure fat; however, of all the commonly used oils, canola oil is the clear winner. Canola oil has half the saturated fat of olive oil or sunflower oil, and has high levels of omega 6 and very high levels of omega 3 fatty acids. These high levels of omega fatty acids may reduce the risk of coronary artery disease, and physicians and dieticians recommend replacing butter, lard, cooking oils and margarine with canola oil and canola oil margarine.

But remember to keep your total fat intake low.

The Bottom Line

There is no question that a low fat diet is healthy. Educate yourself about where the bad fats hide and how to increase the good fats in your diet plan.

Protein

Protein metabolism is extremely important to general health and wellbeing. Muscle, tendon, bone, skin and internal organs are protein; the vital biomolecules hemoglobin, hormones, antibodies and neurotransmitters are proteins. Proteins are huge, 3D molecules made of many building blocks called amino acids. There are over 20 amino acids; most can be made by our cells, but the 9 essential amino acids must come from our diet. Not only must we have an adequate daily supply of protein, but the ratio of amino acids making up the dietary protein must be correct. Humans need quality protein.

- Protein is in a constant state of renewal. Unlike fats and carbs, we can't store protein. We need a steady diet of quality protein or the body breaks down muscle tissue to recycle amino acids.

- Not all dietary protein is created equal. Complete protein has all the amino acids, including the 9 essential amino acids. Incomplete protein doesn't.

- Red meat is a source of complete, high quality protein, iron and vitamins but it is heavy in artery clogging saturated fat. Avoid it.

- Excellent complete protein: skinless poultry, fatty fish, egg whites, nonfat dairy and quinoa.

- Soy protein/tofu/soy milk is complete protein, but questions remain regarding risks for men with the level of plant estrogens in soy.

- Complete protein is especially crucial for athletes, growing adults and pregnant women.

- For vegetarians and vegans, the practice of mixing different types of plant protein is critical. This is referred to as complementary protein mixing, and involves combining two incomplete plant protein sources to mimic the amino acid profile in meat, but without all the saturated fat. See Vegan Issues for more information on this important topic.

- Protein deficiency causes growth failure, weakens immunity and increases risk of injury.

- Excessive protein intake is associated with osteoporosis, bone fractures, liver and kidney problems.

- Estimated daily protein: .4 gm/pound of body weight. This value will vary depending upon activity level, exercise, metabolic rate and other factors.

Phytochemicals

Phytochemicals or phytonutrients are bioactive compounds found in fruits, vegetables, beans, nuts and grains. There are thousands of known phytochemicals and most of their functions are not fully understood as yet. Many, like beta-carotene and resveratrol, have already been linked to significant health benefits. Unlike vitamins, they are not essential for human life but there is compelling evidence that they protect against aging, cancer, heart disease, diabetes and other chronic degenerative diseases.

Prominent Phytochemicals

- Carotenoids – found primarily in yellow, orange and red pigmented plants (carrots, sweet potatoes, pumpkin, tomatoes). Act as antioxidants, support immune system and eye health.

- Flavonoids or Bioflavonoids – large group of compounds that are founds in berries, red grapes, tea, citrus and soy. Act as antioxidants, anti-inflammatory agents and support cardiovascular health.

- Phytosterols – plant derived compounds similar to cholesterol found in nuts, seeds, whole grains and unrefined plant oil. Act to inhibit cholesterol absorption.

- Phytoestrogens – plant derived compounds similar to estrogen found primarily in soy products. Have estrogen-like activities that may protect against certain cancers.

- Organosulfur compounds – found primarily in garlic and onions. Act as antioxidants, anti-inflammatory agents, reduce cholesterol production, support cardiovascular health and reduce risk of certain types of cancer.

- Resveratrol – found in grapes, red wine, peanuts and berries. Acts as antioxidant, improves cardiovascular health and reduces risk of certain types of cancer.

Scientific understanding of the role of phytochemicals in fighting human disease is in its infancy and although promising, there is much research yet to be done. One mechanism of action may be by neutralizing harmful free radicals, but other complex pathways are probably also involved. However, there is little doubt that a healthy diet with ample fresh fruits and vegetables results in a significantly lower incidence of disease. Numerous studies have shown that vegetarians are 40% less likely to develop cancer than meat eaters. Plant based diets provide the protective benefits of phytochemicals and fiber without the fat and carcinogens found in red meat. It should be noted that phytochemical supplements or formulations have not been shown to be as effective as actually eating the fruits, vegetables, beans and grains that contain the natural molecules.

Diet and Weight Management

A healthy diet and weight management plan may be the single most important thing you can do for your fitness, longevity and quality of life. Although simple, this requires discipline and dedication as well as a clear understanding of basic nutritional science.

The human body functions like a machine, and weight management is a simple daily equation:

<u>Input (what you eat) - Output (activity) = Change in Weight</u>

- Moderately active males burn 2500 calories per day, females burn 2200. Athletes burn more.

- Eat less than your activity level requires and your body will burn stored carbs and fat for fuel, and you will lose weight.

- Eat more than your activity level requires and the excess will be stored as fat. An extra 3500 calories equals one pound of body fat.

- Basal Metabolic Rate (BMR) – Energy burned by activity. BMR increases with muscle mass, decreases with age.

- Calorie Count – You won't have to count calories forever, but you need to learn the caloric value of the various foods you eat. Keep a journal of everything you put in your mouth for a week; it may surprise you. Once you get a feel for calorie counting, it will become second nature. A glass of wine/beer/cocktail daily equals 15 pounds of fat per year. Google has a quick, easy to use calorie counter.

- Nutrition Facts – The FDA requires this label. Read it on everything you buy. Select the healthiest foods using the label as your guide. Pay attention to: Calories, Protein, Fat (Sat/UnSat), Cholesterol, Trans Fat and especially Fat Calories. Check serving size; labels often show small serving sizes to lower fat/calorie content.

- Frequent Small Meals – There is evidence this eating pattern is healthier than three large meals as it allows a slower, more even absorption of nutrients, avoiding the spikes of sugar that the body sees as excess and stores as fat.

- *Hara Hachi Bu* – Japanese mantra: Eat until <u>mostly</u> full. This culture of restraint helps explain their health and longevity.

- Check weight daily, at the same time each day.

- Regular exercise may be the true miracle cure. Any exercise is good: walking, running, strength training, aerobics. Just 30 minutes daily burns fat, increases metabolic rate, lowers blood pressure, improves blood flow and brain function and may even prevent cancer.

- Miracle fad diets never work. They are short term regimens of unhealthy nutrition, designed to rapidly drop weight. Usually the dieter relapses back to their old eating habits.

- Balanced Diet – Much is made of the Carb/Fat/Protein ratio when discussing diets. Although the guidelines are roughly 45-65% Carb, 10-35% Protein, and 20-35% Fat, there is no perfect ratio. Understand each food group with its benefits and risks, and adjust the ratio to meet your needs.

- Diet for Life: Start a long term plan to improve the quality of your nutrition, and to increase physical activity and exercise.

- One final caveat: It is far easier to avoid gaining weight than it is to shed the weight, once gained.

The Freshman Fifteen

The infamous Freshman Fifteen refers to the sudden, dramatic weight gain that college freshmen typically put on in their first semester and keep through the year. The causes are many: new lifestyles, erratic schedules, buffet style cafeteria lines, dorm life without a kitchen, limited dietary choices, a bounty of sweets and snacks, alcohol, overindulgence, late nights, little exercise and stress. These factors lead to freshmen, especially women, gaining weight at a much faster rate than average Americans.

An Ounce of Prevention Trumps a Pound of Cure

Physicians who treat obesity know it is far easier to put it on than to take it off. While weight loss is certainly possible, a better strategy is to keep the weight off in the first place. Before you indulge, consider that a bag of chips/beer/glass of wine requires 15 minutes on a treadmill to burn off. Moderate your excesses.

Not everyone gains the Freshman Fifteen, but one in three has significant weight gain. Now is the time to understand nutritional science as your diet is totally under your control. Develop and practice a healthy diet based on intelligent eating. Learn the basic principles and continually customize your diet to your own specific needs.

- Understand calorie counts and nutritional labels.

- Frequent small meals.

- Portion control, especially in buffet lines.

- Limit snacks, cookies, junk food, soda, sweets.

- For snacking, eat fresh fruit and vegetables.

- Exercise regularly.

- Moderate alcohol intake – Excessive alcohol intake is a triple threat: empty calories, tendency to eat unwisely while drinking and a craving for greasy food later.

Vegan Issues

A vegan lifestyle may be good for health, animals and the environment, but following a vegan diet without education can result in malnutrition and chronic fatigue. Vegetable sources of protein are incomplete, both in quality and quantity of amino acids, especially the essential amino acids. Complementary proteins must be eaten, like rice and beans to mimic red meat. This is especially critical for athletes, childbearing age women and growing adults. Vegans can suffer from protein, iron, Vitamin B12 and calcium deficiencies. Before beginning a vegan diet, be sure that you understand the scientific principles of nutrition, protein metabolism and mineral and vitamin requirements and can balance protein sources.

Complementary Proteins

Humans require dietary protein in order to make the muscle, biomolecules, hemoglobin, neurotransmitters and enzymes key to metabolism. Amino acids are the building blocks of protein, and while many of the amino acids we need can be synthesized in the cell, there are 9 essential amino acids that we cannot make. These amino acids must be present in our diet, and ingested on a daily basis as we cannot store protein like we can store fat and carbohydrates. The daily protein requirement is further complicated by the fact that we need our amino acids in a specific ratio to each other, in essence the same ratio found in red meat. With the single exception of quinoa, all plant protein sources are incomplete, meaning they are lacking in the essential amino acids and that the ratio of the other amino acids is suboptimal. Furthermore, the amino acid profile of human protein is different from that of plant protein. These facts, taken together, make complementary protein mixing critical.

Complementary protein mixing has been practiced for centuries by cultures with limited meat in their diets; the classic form is rice and beans. The key element is to mix two incomplete proteins, thereby mimicking the complete protein profile of meat. So while rice is lacking in the amino acid lysine, beans are high in lysine and the result is a meal that supplies the required quantity of amino acids in the required, correct ratio. The complementary proteins must be taken together, preferably at the same time to maximize protein synthesis. Anyone adhering to a vegan or vegetarian diet must understand and practice complementary protein mixing to maintain a healthy, balanced protein metabolism.

Beware: Misinformation abounds on this topic.

Go to reliable, medical sources for education, such as www.nutrition.gov.

Vitamin D

Vitamin D regulates calcium uptake and bone formation, but is not truly a vitamin because it can be synthesized in our skin when exposed to adequate sunlight. In the 19th century, it was discovered that a Vitamin D deficiency caused rickets, a childhood bone disease; the introduction of Vitamin D fortified milk virtually eliminated the disease. However, recent epidemiological evidence and cellular research point to a widespread Vitamin D deficiency with significant new health risks. Just as rickets was seen in the dark, overcast and sooty northern cities during the Industrial Revolution, Vitamin D deficiency is now being seen in our modern, indoor, sedentary population. Video games instead of outdoor activities, our indoor work environment, the use of sunscreen and a general decline in sun exposure have led to a silent epidemic of Vitamin D deficiency.

Vitamin D deficiency increases the risk of depression, bone disease, osteoporosis, heart disease, obesity, breast cancer and prostate cancer. The breakthrough discovery that Vitamin D is essential in activating the immune system's killer T cells may explain the increased incidence of the common cold during winter, as well as the protective effect of Vitamin D in certain cancers. More study of Vitamin D is needed, but this is a very promising field in medical research.

Vitamin D Supplements

Vitamin D is found in very few foods: salmon and fatty fish, egg yolks, fortified milk and fortified cereals. And while it is available free from the sun with ten minutes of skin exposure every other day, the risk of skin cancer must be considered. Furthermore, dark skin tones, cloudy days, clothing and windows all act to block skin synthesis. Studies show that 77% of American adults are deficient in Vitamin D. Experts recommend a Vitamin D3 supplement to assure healthy blood levels year round.

Recommended Adult Dose Vitamin D3 600 IU/Day

Warning: Vitamin D is fat soluble, therefore any excess will accumulate in adipose tissue. Overdosage is possible, and intake of more than 4000 IU/day is dangerous and may result in hypercalcemia, kidney stones and kidney disease.

A Simple Healthy Diet

A twenty-year study[7] of the rural Chinese diet found that a plant based diet with minimal animal products results in a lower incidence of heart disease, cancer, diabetes and obesity. The authors of the study suggest that a plant based diet contains a large number of antioxidants, fiber and nutrients that will promote good health while the animal based diet contains fat and disease producing toxins. While there are factors other than diet in the China study, such as genetics and cultural influences, the conclusions are hard to ignore. Numerous books have been written on the virtues of a low fat, vegetarian diet and its positive effects on heart disease and diabetes. It may be difficult to eat the rural Chinese diet in the US, but following these simple guidelines has been shown to improve health:

- Eat foods as close to the source as possible. Avoid highly processed and preserved food. Organic fruits and vegetables have no pesticides. Free range animals are less fatty than grain feed animals. The best fish is wild salmon, halibut, cod or sole. Nuts (walnuts, Brazil nuts, hazelnuts, almonds) provide a healthy source of protein and fiber.

- Avoid "bad" carbs: white bread, white rice, high fructose corn syrup and sugar. They are refined carbohydrates with a high glycemic index.

- Eat "good" carbs: whole wheat bread, whole-wheat pasta, brown rice, nuts, fruits and vegetables. They are high in fiber with a low glycemic index.

- Avoid saturated fats and trans fats. Most saturated fats come from animal products such as meat and whole milk. Trans fats are found in baked goods, margarines, snack foods and fried food. Avoid or limit fried foods, cream sauces, mayo, butter, cakes, cookies, donuts, chips and processed foods.

- Drink water and tea. Green tea has the most antioxidants and the lowest caffeine. Never drink "fruit drinks"; they have a high glycemic index and added sugar/ high fructose corn syrup. Drink fruit juice (100% juice with no added sugar) occasionally as they too have a high glycemic index. It is always better to eat the actual fruit.

- Do not overeat; eat until you feel just sated. There is a thirty minute delay before your brain senses gastric fullness; the extra food consumed during that half hour becomes fat.

---

7 Campbell, T. Colin, and Campbell, Thomas M. *The China Study: The Most Comprehensive Study of Nutrition Ever Conducted and the Startling Implications for Diet, Weight Loss and Long-term Health.* BenBella Books, 2006.

- Abstain from alcohol, or drink in moderation (2 drinks per day/men, 1 drink per day/women). Choose beer or wine, avoid hard alcohol. Vitamin B6 in beer lowers the blood homocysteine level, which has been linked to heart disease. Wine contains phytochemicals (flavonoids and resveratrol) whose antioxidant properties reduce cell damage and lower LDL cholesterol levels. Recent studies suggest that red or purple grape juice accomplishes the same health benefit as red wine.

- Exercise regularly and take a multivitamin.

High Fructose Corn Syrup (HFCS)

High fructose corn syrup (HFCS) may kill you, literally. First synthesized by chemists from corn syrup in the 1950s as a cheap way to sweeten foods, HFCS is a preservative and a highly concentrated form of fructose. Far cheaper than table sugar, HFCS is everywhere: soft drinks, candy, juices, jams and jellies, flavored yogurt, breads, cereals and many other processed foods like pasta sauces and ketchup. Consumption in the US has skyrocketed to 70 pounds per capita in 2005, by some estimates 17% of our total energy intake. Researchers feel that this fructose overload may be causing our epidemic of obesity and increasing the risk of Type II diabetes, cancer, kidney failure, hypertension and cardiovascular disease. Recent studies at Princeton University strongly implicate HFCS in obesity, and the research continues. Without question, too much HFCS is unhealthy.

Factors Implicating HFCS in the Obesity Epidemic:

• The huge volume of HFCS consumed by Americans.

• Fructose is metabolized differently by the liver than other simple sugars. Rather than being used efficiently for fuel or stored as glycogen like glucose, the fructose pathway produces fatty acids, elevating serum triglycerides and resulting in body fat deposition much like the saturated fat in red meat does.

• Rising levels of fructose in the blood do not stimulate the release of insulin or leptin, like glucose does. This means you do not feel full after eating HFCS sweetened foods; your body does not get the signal to stop eating and you tend to overeat and your metabolism slows.

Eliminating HFCS from Your Diet

Start reading the Nutrition Facts label and Ingredient List on all food you buy, looking for HFCS. Avoid any product where it is listed as an ingredient, especially if high on the ingredient list. Cut back on your refined, simple sugar intake. Replace soda and syrupy juices with pure unsweetened juices or water. Minimize sweets and sugary kid's cereals. By avoiding HFCS, you can drop over 300 calories per day, or over 30 pounds per year from your diet, decrease your body fat percentage, and live a longer, healthier life.

Diet Tricks

Eating is fun. Eating ranks very highly in our list of pleasurable activities, and it is also something we have to do to survive. So cutting into that pleasure, either to lose weight or to manage our health, can be a challenge. Here are techniques that make this struggle palatable:

• Eat a good breakfast within 1h of waking. Carb plus protein is best.

• A light cardio workout, even just a brisk 10 minute walk, will jack up your BMR for the entire day.

• Five small meals are better than three large meals.

• Small meals, small portions.

• Lunch should be small with protein and complex carbs to keep glucose stable, and a little fat to give satiety.

• Fifteen minutes before dinner, drink a Low Sodium V8® vegetable juice or smoothie to reduce hunger and decrease total food ingested.

• Avoid drinking anything with dinner. Fluids dilute enzymes and impair digestion. Alcohol (1 drink) may be beneficial, but is empty calories at about 150 cal/glass of wine, and other foods can provide same benefit.

• Drink ice water and a slice of citrus instead of alcohol, soda, sports drinks, juices, etc.

• Add fiber to all meals; it has no calories but great benefits. Fiber gives volume to food, increases the feeling of fullness and is healthy for your digestive system. Go slowly initially as your system adjusts to the fiber.

• Take your time. Enjoy the meal. Eat slowly. The stomach takes 20-30 minutes to realize it is full, and turn off the hunger drive. This is a major cause of overeating in the US; conversely, the leisurely social atmosphere associated with eating in Europe may be one of the reasons for the much lower obesity rates there.

• Put your fork down until the food in your mouth is thoroughly chewed and swallowed. This maximizes the nutritive quality of the food, especially protein, and assures that all the nutrients are fully absorbed by the body.

• Prepare small healthy portions of fish/chicken/meat and freeze for easy preparation with fresh vegetables/salad/pasta to control portion size.

• Portion Size – An adequate, healthy meat or fish portion size for an adult is approximately the size of a deck of playing cards.

Nutrition Facts

Serving Size 1 packet (40g/1.41 oz)
Servings Per Container 8

Amount Per Serving

Calories 150   Calories from Fat 25

% Daily Value*

Total Fat 2.5g	**4**%
Saturated Fat 0g	**0**%
Trans Fat 0g	
Polyunsaturated Fat 1g	
Monounsaturated Fat 0.5g	
Cholesterol 0mg	**0**%
Sodium 0mg	**0**%
Total Carbohydrate 27g	**9**%
Dietary Fiber 4g	**16**%
Soluble Fiber 1g	
Sugars less than 1g	
Protein 6g	

Vitamin A 0%	•	Vitamin C 0%
Calcium 2%	•	Iron 8%

*Percent Daily Values are based on a 2,000 calorie diet. Your daily values may be higher or lower depending on your calorie needs:

		Calories:	2,000	2,500
Total Fat	Less than		65g	80g
Sat Fat	Less than		20g	25g
Cholesterol	Less than		300mg	300mg
Sodium	Less than		2,400mg	2,400mg
Total Carbohydrate			300g	375g
Dietary Fiber			25g	30g

Calories per gram:
Fat 9 · Carbohydrate 4 · Protein 4

Nutritional Facts: Oatmeal

FDA Nutrition Facts Label

The federally mandated Nutrition Facts label is an excellent consumer aid and health guide. It allows assessment of individual products, and comparison of similar products. It should be studied before you buy any product. Healthy nutrition starts at the grocery store.

Note: Nutrition Facts should be reviewed on everything you consume, and you should keep a running account in your head of your daily consumption.

How to Read the Label www.fda.gov

Serving Size/Serving Number – This is the first step. Often deceptively small serving sizes are used to minimize fat and calorie values; i.e. a small potato chip bag may claim to have three servings, or a cookie bag claim that one cookie is a serving. Determine what you consider a serving, and then calculate the true nutritional values.

Calories – See how the calorie count fits with your daily needs.

Calories from Fat – This is crucial. Fat calories should be limited and not exceed 30% of total caloric input per day.

The rest of the Nutrition Facts label assumes a 2000 calorie daily diet.

Total Fat – Should be low in packaged food. Get your healthy fats from fresh foods and fish. Consider not only the amount of fat intake, but also the types of fats consumed.

• Saturated Fat – Aim for zero here, or the lowest possible number.

• Trans Fat – Zero. There should be no trans fat in your diet.

• Monounsaturated Fat (MUFA) – Healthy fat, lowers cholesterol.

• Polyunsaturated Fat (PUFA) – Healthy fat, lowers cholesterol.

Cholesterol – Limit this nutrient. Low cholesterol diets are healthy.

Sodium – Limit salt to 2000mg/d if healthy, 1500mg/d if hypertensive.

Total Carbohydrate – Total Carb load.

• Dietary Fiber – High values are good.

• Sugars – High values are bad.

Protein – Total protein in the serving.

Vitamins – Critical vitamins supplied in the serving.

Scan the entire label. If the numbers are wrong, find another product. Within a short time you will find the products and brands that have the taste you enjoy with the nutrition you demand.

Ingredient List

The other federally mandated label on foods is the Ingredient List. This lists all ingredients in a food product <u>in order by weight</u>, with the major ingredient first. Make a habit of reading the ingredient list of every single food item you buy. What you will learn will be enlightening, and often surprising. Understanding fully what is in food products allows you to make healthy choices, and to be an intelligent consumer. Avoid any foods with these ingredients, especially if they are one of the first four ingredients in the list:

• High fructose corn syrup (also called corn sugar)

• Corn syrup

• Fruit juice concentrate, maltose, dextrose, sucrose (added sugars)

• Tropical oils (coconut oil, palm oil, palm kernel oil)

• Artificial sweeteners

• Butter

Super Foods

Foods you should include in your diet, with their associated beneficial nutrients:

• Oranges and Citrus Fruits – Vit C, fiber, folate.

• Apples – Vit C, soluble fiber.

• Whole Grain Breads – Fiber, wheat germ, complex carbs.

• Cantaloupe – Vit A, Vit C, carotenoids.

• Broccoli – Vit C, carotenoids, fiber, folate.

• Sweet Potato – Vit C, carotenoids, folate, fiber, Vit K.

• Fat-Free, Skim, Low-fat Milk or Chocolate Milk – Calcium, protein, carbs.

• Red Beans and Kidney Beans – Protein, folate, iron, fiber.

• Salmon, Swordfish, Tuna, Trout – Omega 3 fats, high grade protein.

• Bran Cereal: Kellogg's All Bran Original or Post 100%Bran – Fiber.

• Spinach or Kale – Vit C, carotenoids, calcium, fiber.

• Tomato, Tomato Sauce (if cooked with fat) – Lycopene.

• Peanut Butter – Heart healthy monounsaturated fat, protein.

• Almond Butter – Heart healthy monounsaturated fat, protein.

• Watermelon – Vit K, Vit C, carotenoids.

• Butternut Squash – Vit A, Vit C, fiber, carotenoids.

• Brown Rice, Basmati Rice – Fiber, complex carbs.

• Walnuts, Brazil Nuts and Almonds – Protein, Omega 3 fats.

• Berries: Blueberries, Blackberries, Strawberries – Antioxidants.

• Quinoa – Excellent plant source of high quality protein, fiber.

• Hard Boiled Egg Whites – Perfect source of complete protein.

• Non-fat Ricotta Cheese – protein source (whey).

• Non-fat Yogurt, Greek Yogurt – Protein, calcium, probiotics.

• Flaxseed – Omega 3 fats, fiber.

• Canola Oil – Heart healthy fats for cooking, salads, flavor.

• Oatmeal – Whole grain source of fiber and complex carbs.

• Wheat germ – Fiber, protein, complex carbs, Vit E, antioxidants.

- Carrots – Fiber, carotenoids.
- Lentils – Protein, fiber, Vit B, iron.
- Cruciferous Vegetables: Cauliflower, Cabbage, Broccoli, Brussels Sprouts, Turnips – Soluble Fiber, Vit C.
- Green Tea – Antioxidants.
- Dark Chocolate – Antioxidants, use in small amounts, high in fat.
- Vegetable Juice, V8® – Lycopene, Vit A, Vit C, Vit E.
- Purple Grape Juice – Has same anti-oxidant benefits as red wine and is healthier.

The Superfood Quinoa (*keen-wah*)

"While no single food can supply all of the essential life-sustaining nutrients, quinoa comes as close as any other in the vegetable or animal kingdom."[8]

Cultivated in the Andes for millennia and called the "mother grain" by the Inca, this ancient crop is so nutritionally complete that NASA has considered it as a long term, sustainable food source for space travel. Commonly thought to be a grain, it is actually the seed of a mountain plant similar to spinach and beets. Quinoa is cooked like rice and has a mild flavor and texture similar to couscous or pasta. Especially beneficial for vegans, vegetarians and those following a heart healthy or gluten-free diet, it is the only plant source of complete, high quality protein. Rich in protein, complex carbs, fiber, minerals and healthy fats, quinoa may actually be the perfect food.

---

8 Philip White, "Nutrient Content and Protein Quality of Quinua and Canihua, Edible Seed Products of the Andes Mountains."

Unhealthy Foods

Foods that increase risk of disease or cancer and should be avoided:

- Processed Meats – Hot dogs, brats, deli meats, cold cuts, ham and bacon. All have nitrites which may cause cancer.

- Fried Foods – Fries, onion rings, fried zucchini, hush puppies, deep fried anything.

- Red Meat – High levels of saturated fat.

- Whole Dairy – High levels of saturated fat.

- Cookies – Pure sugar and fat with no nutritive value.

- Typical Canned Soups – Loaded with salt.

- Ice Cream – Loaded with fat and sugar.

- Soda – Leaches calcium from bones, decalcifies teeth. High in HFCS.

- Sports Drinks – High in sugar and HFCS.

- Flavored Yogurt – Fruit added varieties are heavy with HFCS.

- Chips and Crackers – High levels of trans fat and even low fat varieties have a high glycemic load.

EXERCISE

"Physical fitness is not only one of the most important keys to a healthy body; it is the basis of dynamic and creative intellectual activity."

John Fitzgerald Kennedy 1917-1963

The Basics

Over 70% of Americans are obese or overweight, due to our sedentary lifestyle. Obesity is a major factor in diabetes, heart disease, stroke and arthritis. Diet alone will not reverse these health problems; exercise must be incorporated into your lifestyle. Just 30 minutes of exercise every other day has profound health benefits: longer life span, enhanced self-image, less stress, higher basal metabolic rate (BMR), a leaner more muscular body, lower blood pressure, increased serotonin and endorphin levels, improved memory and brain function, even protection against diabetes and cancer.

- Check with your physician or orthopedic surgeon before starting an exercise program. Go slowly.

- Any and all exercise is good. Walk a mile or run a mile, either works. Take the stairs, walk to lunch, park further away. Do anything but sit.

- Moderate exercise 30 min/5x weekly can melt away the invisible, toxic visceral fat. Visceral fat is stored within the abdomen, is denser and firmer than body fat, and is formed from saturated fat in your diet. It is metabolized into cholesterol by the liver and has been implicated in heart disease, stroke, dementia and diabetes.

- Exercise not only burns fat while you are working out, but causes an elevation of your MR for up to 12 hours afterwards, continuing the fat burning effect.

- The optimal workout program combines aerobic training with strength training. Do not neglect strength training; incorporate some weight or resistance workout into your schedule at least twice a week.

No Pain, No Gain = No Brain

Forget the old saying: "No pain, no gain." It is not only dead wrong, it is dangerous. Pain is your body's way of telling you to stop before injury occurs. Be especially careful of loading or stressing your spine and your joints. Asymptomatic injuries often occur, and can lead to a lifetime of arthritis, pain or disability.

153

Cardio

Cardiovascular, or aerobic workouts are exercises that raise the heart rate to 60-85% of your maximum heart rate for 30-60 min. At this pace you can talk, but can't carry on a conversation easily. This has been proven to burn fat and enhance cardiovascular health. A typical cardio workout is running, jogging, biking, treadmill, rowing, aerobics, even dancing. Heart rate monitors are useful to train effectively and safely.

Recommendation: 30 Minutes Cardio Daily.

Cardio has multiple, far reaching health benefits:

- Burns fat, lowers weight and lowers blood pressure.

- Lowers risk of stroke, diabetes, heart disease.

- Reduces stress, improves sleep.

- Does not increase muscle mass.

Pearls and Principles

Stay hydrated. Breathe deeply. Oxygen is the limiting factor here. Don't worry about time, five minutes is better than nothing, and any exercise is better than no exercise. Have fun. Listen to your iPod. Do what you like. Get proper gear for your training. Go slowly. Don't overdo.

Try Interval Training – Alternating bursts of high intensity intervals with low intensity recovery intervals. Sprint for 1 minute, then jog for 3 minutes. This training method magnifies results significantly.

Shoes – Buy the right shoes for your purpose and terrain. Replace insole with a quality gel sport insole. Well fit, quality shoes minimize injury to your back and knees. There should be at least ½ inch between toes and shoe. Shoes have a lifespan; replace them often.

Change It Up – Try Tae Bo®, Denise Austin, Zumba or P90X® to keep it fun.

Strength Training

A healthy balanced diet and cardio are important, but strength training will increase muscle mass, strengthen bones and improve the look of your body. By increasing muscle mass, you increase your basal metabolic rate (BMR) and burn fat even when you are resting. This is the key to long term weight control. Strength training with weights, resistance or isometrics is essential for a complete exercise program. Consult your physician before beginning any strength training program.

The Basics		
Heavy Weights	1-6 Reps	Strength
Moderate Weights	7-12 Reps	Body Building
Light Weights	13+Reps	Fitness

Pearls and Principles

Aim for a minimum of two workouts per week.

Always start a workout with a 10 minute warm up and end with a cool down and stretches.

The optimal workout combines aerobics and weights. It has been shown that running or cardio should be done <u>after</u> weight lifting to maximize results.

Breathe properly. <u>EXonEX</u>: Exhale on the exertion phase of the exercise. Inhale at the start, exhale during the exertion, inhale again as you return to the starting position. Don't hold your breath or valsalva; this spikes blood pressure dangerously and slows blood return to the heart and lungs.

Proper form is critical. Don't swing weights or let gravity help. Count: 1-2-3 on the lift, 3-2-1 on the lower. Go slow.

Use light weights with high repetitions when beginning. Progressively increase the weight to challenge muscle.

<u>Never load your spine</u>. Keep legs bent. Avoid any exercise that transmits loads, especially vertically, on vertebrae.

Use caution with gym machines. Some are harmful to your joints, tendons and ligaments, such as leg presses and behind the neck lat pulldowns.

Free weights force you to use core and limb muscles for balance, and have more benefit than machines.

Mix whole body exercises and isolated muscle exercises. Whole body exercises like the Lunge/Press strengthen core muscles, improve balance and have cardiovascular benefits.

Change it up. Often. There are many variables you can play with: weight, sets, reps, pyramids, splits, rest periods. Boredom causes plateaus in muscle growth. There is no magical, set in stone formula. Keep it fun.

Medical Alert: The Dangers of Heavy Weights

Remember: You can build muscle, but you <u>cannot</u> strengthen joints; the knee, elbow, hip and shoulder joints are fragile and easily injured by the kind of heavy abnormal loading often seen in body building and weight training. Once damaged, repair is difficult if not impossible, and you will have a lifetime of pain, arthritis, sleep disturbances and diminished function. Heavy weights should be avoided; equivalent results are easily obtained with lighter weights and higher repetitions of proper form.

Always end a workout with a cool down and stretch. This elongates muscle fibers and maximizes repair.

Rest and Repair: To build optimal growth, muscle needs time. Rest at least 48 hours between workouts, and be sure to get a minimum of 8 hours healthy sleep.

Muscle Physiology

There are two types of muscle: slow twitch (Type I) for endurance, and fast twitch (Type II) for speed and power. Studies show that training alters the ratio of these fibers in athletes, so train for your specific sport.

Exercise causes microtears in the muscle that must be repaired to grow. High quality protein must be provided to the healing muscle along with carbs to recharge glycogen stores. For 30 minutes after a hard workout, the channels are open wide in muscle cells to replenish glycogen and rebuild muscle. After 30 minutes, the process continues, but at a far slower rate. Be sure to have a small protein/carb post workout meal.

Sports Nutrition

Sports drinks, performance enhancers and nutritional supplements are a $6 billion industry, based largely on hype.

Hydrate – Water hydrates without added calories that can negate your entire workout. Avoid juices and sports drinks that often contain HFCS. Avoid colas, coffee, sodas with caffeine. In long runs, especially in hot climates, dehydration can cause sludging of blood and negate your exercise benefits. Stay ahead of your thirst.

Sports drinks – Rarely necessary in workouts <1hour. In strenuous workouts >1hour, a 6% carb plus electrolyte sports drink may help rehydration. In long endurance events, a 4:1 carb:protein drink may speed muscle recovery, store glycogen and help the immune system.

Alcohol – Retards muscle development, depresses growth hormone and testosterone, and slows recovery. Toxic to muscle.

NSAIDs – Non Steroidal Anti-Inflammatory Drugs: aspirin, ibuprofen, naprosyn, etc. Excellent drugs for minor pains; but by blunting inflammation, they stop muscle repair, and negate your workout progress by inhibiting growth of new muscle.

Training Table

If you eat like a NFL lineman, you will soon look like one. Muscle is built in milligram increments, not by the pound. Overdoing it at the training table is not only unhealthy, it reverses any positive effect in body sculpting and lean muscle mass that you have worked so hard to achieve. To optimize your results:

Before Workout

- Light protein/carb meal 2 hours before working out.
- Green Tea – Shown to increase endurance.
- Hydrate – Preload with water 1 hour before working out.

During Workout

- Maintain hydration – Keep ahead of thirst with water or diluted sports drink.

Post Workout

- Recharge within 30 minutes – Carbs plus quality protein. Low fat chocolate milk is perfect. Milk is an excellent source of protein, and the chocolate has antioxidants for muscle repair. Ratio 4:1 carb:protein. Too much protein is actually harmful and delays regeneration.

Protein Supplements

- Whey – Fast acting, quickly absorbed milk protein. This is perfect for immediately after a workout; shown to increase muscle synthesis.

- Casein – Slow acting milk protein. Excellent for the 48 hours of repair when muscle is being slowly rebuilt. Perfect for a bedtime smoothie.

- Quinoa – Complete, high quality plant protein source. Now farmed on small scale in South America. This grain holds great promise in future.

- Soy – Plant protein with phytoestrogens, whose hormonal effects are not yet clear. Inferior.

Muscle Building Supplements

There are hundreds of expensive and ineffective products claiming to enhance muscle development, increase energy or strength and give you the 'edge'. Avoid these supplements. You can get everything you need to build muscle in the healthy diet outlined here.

Medical Alert: Performance Enhancing Supplements

There are many legal and illegal supplements available, and a huge underground industry providing steroids, growth hormone, DHEA, testosterone precursors, prohormones, creatine and other ways to 'boost' performance. Growth hormone is extremely dangerous, creatine has been linked to kidney failure and testosterone and steroids cause permanent facial disfigurement and disease. In healthy athletes, all that is needed is disciplined training and balanced nutrition.

PERSONAL SAFETY

"Know safety, no injury..
No safety, know injury."

Anonymous

The Vigilant Philosophy

Your personal safety is your responsibility and yours alone. Despite the rhetoric, the police cannot protect you at any given moment, nor is it their duty. In reality, you are simply on your own. The police, at best, may apprehend the criminal after the crime. Even with the finest protection in the world, heavily armed Secret Service agents, our Presidents have been shot by determined assassins.

Prevention and avoidance is by far the best strategy for personal safety. Self-defense isn't about fighting; it's about avoiding conflict by using your brain, not your fists. Your behavior affects your personal safety, from how you walk on the sidewalk, to your transactions at the grocery store. You must cultivate and practice a lifelong state of vigilance.

Depending on our age, stature, fitness and mental attitude, we all develop our own self preservation system. Martial arts are effective, but require daily practice and tremendous discipline and physical prowess. And in real world fights, there are no winners.

- Remember material goods should always be forfeited for personal health; in other words, give up your wallet or purse rather than fight and be injured. Take the time now to "back up" your wallet or purse as described later in this section. This "back up" renders your actual wallet inconsequential, and makes surrendering it far easier.

- Avoidance, de-escalation and retreat are not cowardice. Live to fight another day.

- Fight only as an absolute last resort.

- Body Language – You are either predator…or prey. This is how criminals assess you. An aware, confident look or posture, even just having a whistle on your keychain may deter attack.

360° Situational Awareness

When you observe animals in the wild, they are hyperaware of their surroundings. Constantly looking, smelling, listening, sensing. For 21st century Americans, the risk from lions, tigers and bears is negligible. The risk from predatory humans is very real. Situational awareness is essential.

Backing Up Your Wallet and Keys

- Make your wallet or purse easily replaceable by backing up your information, just as you would on your computer. Copy your driver's license, credit cards and club cards (SSN, health club, warehouse memberships, AAA) and keep them secure.

- Never put your Social Security card in your wallet or purse. Memorize your number and lock the card away.

- Make a "call sheet" with phone numbers of your credit card companies, DMV, club memberships, etc. to call immediately if your wallet or purse is stolen or lost.

- Limit personal information in your wallet or purse. If possible, use your parent's home or business address for your driver's license address. Never print your home address or phone number on your checks.

- Keep a separate copy of your car key just for valet service or auto repair shops. Never give a valet or anyone else your full set of keys (auto, home or apartment, work, etc). Criminals can take a wax imprint of a key in seconds, and thereby have access to your home, car and office.

The Buddy System

The buddy system has long been used for safety in the military (wingman), firefighting (two in, two out) and the Boy Scouts (two deep). It works and can be utilized in the college or urban environment. It's about looking out for each other, when you are at a party, running, hiking or shopping. Having someone with you reduces risk, deters criminals, enables someone to monitor and assist you, all the time allowing you to enjoy your event with good company.

- Choosing your buddy is critical. Does this person share the same ethics and morals as you do? A good friend makes you a better person and steers both of you out of trouble, not into it. Does this person do this? Do you?

- Discuss with your buddy what you expect. Do they have your back? Never leave a buddy stranded, especially when at a party or bar. If your buddy is drunk, take them home. Don't let their altered judgment dictate the day. Be smart, be safe.

- Use the buddy system in bars and party environments. Tell your buddy what you are doing and where you are going. Never leave without your buddy.

- Use your cell phone and internet as your buddy if you are alone. Get a cell phone with a GPS feature and activate it. Email or call a friend and tell them where you are and what you are doing. You can even call or email yourself to document who you are with and where you are going. Authorities can look at your emails and phone messages to help you if necessary.

- Take cell phone photos of your date, license plates, people or places and text message to a friend or family to document your surroundings.

- Let everyone know that you are communicating with a friend or family member (even if you are just sending this to yourself). This is a deterrent to criminals. Most people are harmless, but it is better to be safe than sorry.

Patterned Response

A patterned response is an excellent method for dealing with recurring, normal but annoying situations in everyday life. These things happen over and over, and your response is always the same, e.g.: street people, panhandlers, telephone solicitation, unwanted romantic overtures, door to door salesmen, petition drives and so on. Having a rehearsed and ready reply to these approaches closes the matter quickly, keeps their foot out of the door, and saves time and face. This is especially important in romantic advances, as a rude response may beget an angry reaction. Practice with a friend until the patterned response is natural.

Romantic Advance:	*You are gorgeous. Can I take you to dinner?*
You:	*Thank you, but I have a boyfriend/girlfriend.*
	I'm married/in a committed relationship.
High Pressure Salesperson:	*You need to pay an extra $500 for that.*
You:	*Let me discuss this with my spouse/lawyer/accountant.*
	I will consider it and get back with you.
	I don't think so.
Telemarketer:	*Is this Jane Doe?*
You:	*Who is calling? What can I do for you?*
	I am not interested.
	Please add me to your "Do Not Call List". Thank you.
Stranger/Panhandler:	*Spare change? Can you help me?*
You:	*No, thank you. (An illogical response that is the nicest way to say no. Ends the dialogue.)*

The key in all patterned responses is that it be non-confrontational, polite, and brief but final.

The Sociopath, Psychopath, or Antisocial Personality

These three terms are used interchangeably, and refer to a spectrum of abnormal and destructive behavior ranging from deceit and habitual lying to animal cruelty, rape or serial murder. It is estimated that 5% of the population exhibits this behavior, and you will certainly encounter them. This section is not meant to diagnose or label any individual; it is meant to help you identify and avoid sociopaths. The ability to recognize and avoid a sociopath is invaluable.

Characteristics

The common unifying traits are: constant lying, complete lack of conscience, guilt or responsibility and selfishness and disregard for consequences. They live in the moment.

• Sociopaths do not feel emotion deeply; their "feelings" are just shallow displays for secondary benefit.

• They are totally amoral with no conscience. They have no empathy for those they damage. No remorse.

• Dishonesty. Expert and habitual liars. Eloquent and persuasive. Seductive.

• Socially adept: interesting, charming, "life of the party", center of attention, eager to please. Outwardly seem successful and competent. Often weave a complex imaginary world that is real to them.

• Dreamers without commitment: grandiose schemes, investments and plans, but no responsibility.

• When confronted, rationalize or redirect. Never accept responsibility.

• Often the last one you would suspect. Deception is elaborate and convincing.

It is not yet known if this behavior is learned or genetic. Studies show that their nervous systems don't react when they lie (no nervousness, sweating, eye tells), making them treacherous. Recognizing a sociopath is difficult; heed the red flags. Realize that if they are lying to others, they will also lie to you. Avoid them as they cannot be changed or cured and often do tremendous personal and financial damage to those around them.

Assault

Violent crime is common in the US, with approximately 17,000 murders and over 200,000 assaults yearly. Martial arts, pepper spray or weapons are more fantasy than reality, and should be used only as the last resort. Often in violent crimes the victims put themselves in the wrong place, at the wrong time. Avoiding trouble is far easier, safer and much wiser.

Trust Your Animal Instincts

Humans have evolved, but still retain primal instincts and can sense danger. Studies show we can smell fear and anger pheromones. We have all experienced it: chills, hair standing on end, heightened senses. If you feel uncomfortable, your instincts are warning you: Beware.

Assess your situation. Never take chances. Use these techniques, and adapt them to your situation:

- Take a class in basic self defense and <u>practice</u>. Master one hard strike.

- Use the buddy system. Never jog or walk alone. If you have to jog and do not have a buddy, go to a gym. Ask for a staff member to walk you to your car when leaving.

- Keep your home safe and secure. Get in the habit of doing a perimeter check: Walk around your home or apartment, securing all windows and doors. Activate alarm if you have one.

- Check ID of service people before allowing entrance. This is a common criminal ruse. If you did not call for a service person, do not open the door or let them in. Tell them through the door that you will need to re-schedule another time. Call their company and verify. Call police if this was not a legitimate service call.

- Avoid isolated areas where there are few people (parking lots, laundry rooms, garages, library-late night, work after-hours).

- Always park near the building in a well-lit area. When possible, park your car with the driver's door facing the building entrance/exit.

- Always have your keys ready when approaching your car or house.

- Look around as you approach your car. Check the back seat before entering.

- Know where the "panic" button is on your car key and test it monthly.

- Do not offer rides to people you do not know well. And never pick up a hitchhiker.

- Avoid drug use or heavy alcohol use. Your judgment and ability to protect yourself will be impaired.

- Always be aware of your surroundings; survey where you are and where you are going.

- Never stop when approached by strangers, panhandlers, etc. Always keep moving. Once you stop, they can get too close and you have the problem of disengaging. Just keep moving.

- Practice screaming, "Leave me alone!" or "Don't touch me!" or "Fire!" SCREAM as loud as you can when necessary. It may save your life. FIGHT! RUN!

- Vary your schedule and routes and routines (lunch/laundry/route to class or work).

- When entering bar/club/party: Scan the room, check for exits, feel and sense if there is an aura of tension. If there is any doubt, leave.

Be careful in locations and situations when you are in increased danger or vulnerability: Getting in/out of cars, standing in doorways, in parking lots, elevators, hotels, darkness, clubs, away from home (vacations), ATMs, public phones and anywhere your attention is diverted. The best prevention for assault is situational awareness and avoidance.

Drug Facilitated Sexual Assault (DFSA) or Date Rape

The incidence of forcible rape, statutory rape, date rape and sexual assault is high. Surveys of college age women show that one in four women has been attacked, often by someone they know. One in ten men is sexually assaulted, but men rarely report the incident. DFSA drugs such as rohypnol, GHB and ketamine are odorless, tasteless and readily available. They have rapid onset, are powerful, and disappear quickly leaving no evidence. These drugs are also used for robbery and assaults. Protect yourself at bars and parties:

- Vigilance is the best defense for women <u>and</u> men.

- Clearly state your limits in all relationships.

- Don't be afraid to say "No!"

- Trust your instincts. If you feel uneasy or uncomfortable, leave immediately.

- Always go out in groups, never alone. Make one person the designated driver and watchdog.

- <u>Watch your drink</u>. Never accept free drinks, drinks on the house or free shots. Never exchange drinks or share drinks.

- Never leave your drink unattended. Never leave your drink on a table when you dance or go to the bathroom. If you do, get a new one.

- Never drink anything from punch bowls or vats, frat party style.

- Never drink anything you did not see prepared. Whenever possible, drink canned or bottled beverages and have them opened before your eyes. Specify that to your server, or go to the bar and observe it yourself. Realize that bartenders in some venues have special bottles, laced with drugs, just for girls they want impaired.

- If you sense something is wrong, tell your friends immediately. Call someone responsible who is <u>not</u> partying with you (family). Call 911. If you suspect that you or a friend has been drugged, go to ER for evaluation and treatment. Do not seek help from bar patrons or your new "friends". They may be the ones drugging you. Do not go outside alone or get some "fresh air" with a stranger.

- Volunteer at a Rape Crisis center to help others and learn.

How to Stay Safe in a Nightclub or Bar

Always use the buddy system (See Buddy System). Select a buddy that you trust and who shares your life philosophy and moral standards. Let your other friends know where you are going.

- Always carry a charged cell phone. Have your local taxi company phone number programmed into your cell phone.

- Stay sober. Keep track of the number of drinks you have. Drink very slowly. Remain in control; your decisions will be intelligent and in your best interest.

- Do not drink hard alcohol. Drink bottled drinks and hold the drink; do not put it down.

- Drugs can be placed in alcoholic drinks, soft drinks, tea, coffee or water. If you suspect tampering with your drink, don't drink it. Never leave your drink unattended; watch your drink and your buddy's drink. If you leave your drink to dance or go to the bathroom, don't drink it. Order another.

- If there is a fight or loud argument, or if the clientele is questionable, leave the bar/club with your buddy. If your buddy does not agree, you have the wrong buddy. Insist that you both leave.

- Avoid the "bad drunk". This may be one of your friends. If so, never go out with a "bad drunk". They attract trouble, are unreliable and can turn on you.

- Never accept a drink from anyone you do not know or trust. Never give any information out to a stranger. Never give full names or phone numbers or business cards. You don't know them and they can find you at work or home by internet search.

- Do not send the wrong message with suggestive clothing or by flirting; this type of behavior casts a wide net. You will attract the wrong people for the wrong reasons.

- Never leave the bar with a stranger.

- Do not argue with friends or strangers in a bar. Concede the point and end the discussion.

- Do not "challenge" or act in a rude manner to a stranger in a bar.

- Have fun, but be in control. Be safe.

Designated Driver (DD)

The designated driver is perhaps the most sensible but underused social innovation of our time. DUI is involved in half of accidents, and DUI related fatalities are on the rise. The minimum cost of a DUI is $10,000; the cost of a motor vehicle accident could be your life.

definition: The designated driver is relied upon to pick up, transport, and return home safely the drinker(s). He must remain stone cold sober. If he fails to do so, he must arrange for and provide safe transport of the group by taxi or other means. It is a serious responsibility.

The designated driver is more than just a chauffeur, but a wingperson as well. The DD is the fully functional, sober one in the club, keeping an eye on the group, the tab, the credit cards and the drinks (see Drug Facilitated Sexual Assault). The modern nightclub scene is rife with scams, billing fraud and identity theft. This is especially true in tourist/vacation destinations. Having a sober watchful eye safeguarding the group is invaluable.

Use your DD as a sounding board for the many brilliant ideas that evolve during a night's partying. Ask "Does (fill in the blank) sound like a good idea to you?" before proceeding.

Pearls and Principles

- Select the DD in advance.

- Cover gas expenses for the DD.

- Reward the DD or rotate the responsibility.

- Patronize establishments with complimentary non-alcoholic beverages for DDs.

- Do not tempt the DD to drink.

- Volunteer often to be the DD.

The use of a DD in no excuse for wild, binge drinking by the group.

Exercise restraint in all drinking.

Alcohol is far and away the most dangerous and destructive form of substance abuse.

Drink responsibly.

Dorm Room

Your new roommate is most likely a fine person; however they may not share your philosophy of personal safety. Worse, they may exhibit behavior that can put you in harm's way.

- Be vocal with your opinion and philosophy of personal safety.
- Remember your room key has been duplicated for college employees and former students.
- Get a new lock, re-key existing lock or install a deadbolt.
- Place an electronic entry alarm on the door.
- Is there a smoke detector? Is it working?
- Locate the closest fire exit. You may have to use it in smoke and the dark.
- Place your flashlight, pepper spray, cell phone, etc. at your bedside.
- Have a first aid kit in your room with a manual for emergencies.
- Never let strangers enter your dorm room.

Document Security

Residence halls and apartments are often less secure than a single family dwelling due to high volume of visitors and use of master keys. Until you own a home, it is wise to keep all precious, irreplaceable items and documents in a safe place. Passports, birth certificates, Social Security cards, diplomas and vehicle titles should be stored in a fireproof, waterproof safe at your parents' home or alternatively in a bank safety deposit box. Safety deposit boxes at your bank are extremely secure, inexpensive ($30/year) and convenient. Replacing these documents can be a nightmare, or impossible.

Home or Apartment Security

- Install a home security system or buy a portable alarm system for your apartment. Alarm systems protect your home against burglary and fire. Post the alarm company decals at all likely points of entry: windows, patio doors, entry door.

- Burglars commonly enter through sliding glass doors and windows. Make sure your locks are sturdy. All outside doors should have dead bolts, sliding glass doors should have locks and/or locking bars, window locks should be burglarproof.

- Outside doors should be solid wood or metal.

- Never tell anyone anything about trips, possessions or personal information. This includes social media and blog updates.

- Keep front doors, garage doors and front windows closed.

- Keep valuables out of sight.

- When traveling, stop the mail, deliveries and the newspaper. Let your trusted neighbors know that you are gone.

- Use automatic timers on lights, TV and music when gone.

- Outdoor lights with motion detectors deter burglars. Light up the outside at night.

- Shred your sensitive papers and anything with your address on it. Break down and remove your address from all boxes and parcels, and shred the address before recycling the box.

- Close window shades at night.

- Never open the door for strangers.

Home Emergency Preparedness

• 3 day supply of non-perishable food and water (1 gallon/person/day).

• Cash and credit card.

• Gas camping stove, can opener, utensils, plates, bowls.

• Flashlights, battery powered radio, phone card, cell phone with extra battery, whistle.

• First aid kit.

• Documents – Copies of driver's license, passport, birth certificate, Social Security card, insurance information, bank account statement, credit card information. Protect them and know where they are. Replacing them is a frustrating nightmare.

• Personal items – Prescription medications, personal hygiene items, extra eyeglasses.

• N95 Dust mask (for birdflu, swineflu, influenza), gloves, multi-tool.

• Plastic garbage bags for waste. Duct tape and plastic sheet for sealing windows or doors.

• Extra car keys.

• Chlorine bleach to disinfect surfaces and water (2 drops per quart).

Identity Theft - Shredding

Most of us cannot believe that someone would actually go through our garbage, but it happens more often than you think, and it is perfectly legal for them to do so. The Supreme Court ruled that your trash is public. Simple solution: Buy a cross cutting shredder. For large quantities of material to be shredded (end of year tax material or cleaning out your <u>locked</u> file cabinet), you can take a large box to shredding companies for disposal. When you use a shredding service, be sure to personally watch your box go into the shredder. <u>Never</u> just give documents to a service for destruction at a later time.

Shred:

- Everything with your name and address.
- Everything with your Social Security number.
- Everything related to your taxes and banking.
- Mailing address labels. Look within the mailer for your name and address in other places.
- All bills (phone, utilities, cable, water, etc.).
- Store credit card receipts (name and partial credit card information).
- All credit card documents.
- Credit card mail "offer" forms.
- All printed email documents.
- All banking documents (checks, notices, statements).
- Tax information and old tax forms.
- School grades and transcripts.
- Travel information, itineraries or receipts.
- Used airline tickets/baggage tags (name and frequent flyer information).
- Any type of ID card.
- Old passports (if expired, shred it).
- Employee information (pay stubs, tax information).
- Computer personal information on CD or floppy.
- Any medical or dental information.
- Last year's calendar, date book, old personal phone book.

Identity Theft - Passwords

- Your password should increase in strength with the sensitivity and value of the website. Any website with financial information or requiring use of a credit card or your personal information demands a high strength password. Forums devoted to pastimes are not as critical.

- Consider using password management software.

- Do not use your birth date, initials, Social Security number, home phone number, words, or a sequence (123456).

- Use at least 8 characters; include numbers, symbols and letters (upper and lower case).

- Never share your password with anyone or login with others present.

- Change your password every 6 months or if you think your security has been breached.

- Never write down your password unless you are locking the document in a safe.

- Change your password if you have used it on any computer other than yours (internet café, friend's house, library). The same goes for unsecured hot spots, WiFi and cell phone access to the internet.

- Never give your password out over the internet.

- Try not to use a personal question that one can easily find out such as mother's maiden name. Use something very personal or make up a unique and unexpected answer to a simple question, such as "What is your favorite sports team?" Your answer "Seahorses".

- Never tell anyone the answers to your personal questions.

- Protect your computer with password entry. Change often.

- Do not let anyone use your computer unless it is in the "guest" mode.

- Create a travel temporary email address when traveling and using public computers.

Your Credit Score

As you establish credit, you build a credit history and a credit score from 300 to 850. The higher the score, the better your credit. A score above 700 is good and scores below 620 are poor. Your credit score has substantial, lifelong impact on your financial health, availability of loans and interest rates. A poor score will cost you money and frustrate your life. A good score will save you money and make life easier.

The Three Main Credit Reporting Agencies Are:

- Equifax (800-685-1111)

- Experian (888-397-3742)

- TransUnion (800-888-4213)

- You can obtain your credit report free, once yearly, at 877-FACTACT.

- The credit report displays a monthly record of your payments, how much debt you have, payment, late payment and delinquent payment history, bankruptcy, federal tax liens and who has inquired about your credit history.

- Good credit remains on your report forever; bad credit for 7 to 10 years.

- Review your credit once a year with a free report from any of the agencies. Personal information and history should be carefully examined. Checking regularly protects you from identity theft.

- The credit-reporting agency must investigate errors in your report upon request. If an error occurs, keep records of the error and your attempts to clear the problem.

- If you are denied credit, it is your right to see your credit report.

- To establish and maintain good credit, you should set limits on your monthly credit card usage, pay bills on time in full with no finance charges, understand your credit card terms, have a minimal number of credit cards, review your statements with receipts and think about your spending limit.

Credit Cards

First and foremost, understand that credit cards typically carry interest rates of 22% or more and should <u>never</u> be used as short term or long term loans. Credit card debt is the #1 cause of bankruptcy in young adults and although there are federal consumer protections, the process of restoring your credit can take years. Common mistakes are to pay only the minimum payment each month, and to underestimate the interest cost. Example: a $1500 flat screen TV paid for at $50/month at 21% interest will take 43 months and cost $2150. Read the terms and conditions (all the fine print) very carefully. Rates can increase and there may be stiff penalties for missed and late payments.

- View your credit and debit cards as cash.

- Obtain two credit cards, one for day-to-day purchases and one for the internet.

- Consider using "Cash Back" credit cards that pay 1-5% cash refunds on purchases. Get cards with no annual fee. Check interest rates carefully.

- Your internet credit card should be used only for online purchases. If stolen or pirated, your day-to-day card can still be used.

- Always fill out receipts completely and sign, do not leave anything blank, put a zero with a slash through the center of the zero on blank lines.

- Always review your statement and call the vendor when in doubt. Credit card fraud can occur with small dollar amounts. Criminals will start with a small charge to see if the card is active.

- Keep your statements and credit card customer service numbers in a fireproof safe or locked file cabinet.

- Keep credit card numbers and PINs confidential. Never give the numbers out to an email or telephone solicitor even if they state they are from the credit card company (tell them you will call them back and then call the number on your statement).

- Know when your credit card bill is coming and call the bank if it is late. Your bill has very sensitive data.

- Shred <u>all</u> credit card solicitations.

Shopping Online

- Shop <u>only</u> at reputable, known internet businesses.

- Enter credit card information to websites with "https://" only, which stands for HyperText Transfer Protocol Secure. Non-secure websites are http://.

- Use well known computer security programs such as McAfee, Kaspersky or Symantec.

- Never give any information to a company through an email. Call them if they are asking for information. Confirm the phone number given in your email with the real phone number.

- Designate one credit card for internet transactions only. This way, if you have a problem or the card is pirated, you can then quickly cancel this card without affecting your daily use of your other credit card. You can examine your statement easily for internet fraud.

- Never use a debit or ATM card for internet purchases. This gives criminals access to your bank account. And while credit card companies usually provide protection from fraudulent charges, banks will hold you responsible for any fraudulent charges arising from debit or ATM cards.

- Look for the Better Business Bureau seal of approval for any online business and check their rating at <u>www.BBBonline.org</u>.

- Make sure the site is encrypted (yellow padlock symbol will appear).

- Go to the site with your browser. Never use email solicitations with hyperlinks.

- Consider shipping charges vs. tax, etc. Are you saving money by purchasing online? Always check the return policy prior to buying.

- Avoid online gambling, poker or sports book sites. In case of a dispute, you have little recourse and cashing out your balance can be frustrating.

- Beware of purchasing and giving gift cards. Gift cards are nothing more than unsecured, interest free loans to the store issuing them. They can be lost, stolen, expire or become worthless if the store fails. Cash or a check is always a better gift.

Internet Dating 1

Internet dating is a new and very popular phenomenon, and a perfectly acceptable way to meet quality people. If you decide to pursue internet dating, it is like any dating situation; you must use common sense and protect yourself. All these rules apply to both men and women.

Your Internet Dating Profile and Photos

Profile – This should tell something about you, your interests, but <u>not</u> about your identity. No personal details of job, home or school. No Facebook, blog or social media links.

Photos – Casual attire, not risqué, and no background clues to home, work, school or job. Do not expose yourself to ID theft or stalking.

Internet Correspondence

- Never use your real name/DOB/job in your profile or email address. Establish an alias and <u>forgettable</u> email address just for dating. Use a false birthday, age, job and town. Variations of the truth work well.

- Do all dating correspondence from your dating email account <u>only</u>.

- Use a good chat engine to IM initially. Yahoo has an excellent free platform that allows you to talk via mic, share photos without downloading them (and viruses), and use a webcam.

- You can learn a great deal about someone just by chat. Get to know them. Be sure they have posted many recent photos.

- Get a webcam. They are cheap, fun and will save you many disappointments. Be wary of anyone who will not get a $15 webcam so you can see and talk with them live, as they really are.

- Keep it polite. If it sours, <u>do not flame</u> (rude or angry reply). Just disappear.

Telephone Contact

- After chatting, consider talking by phone. IM chat is imperfect. You can learn much more from a real conversation. Get a cheap disposable cell phone or give your cell number, not your home phone. Spend some time talking, honestly. Block your number with *67.

- Continue to maintain your privacy. No personal details.

- Red Flags: Never answers calls. Always goes to voicemail. Only talks at certain hours. Inconsistencies from profile. Blocked numbers. Whispering. Voices in background. Hanging up. These could mean they are married, have relationship, live at home, are underage, institutionalized or incarcerated.

Internet Dating 2

The First Meeting

This is not a traditional date where you know the person from school, work or friends. It is a meeting with a total stranger. The reality is that the police can trace you both by IP address and cell phone call history, but some criminals don't realize this or don't care. Continue to protect your safety, identity and personal details.

- Remember: This is not a "date". It is not even a blind date. Do not plan for dinner, a movie and drinks. It should be planned to be short (5-30 min) and sweet. The sole purpose of this is to see if the person is anything like their profile, and if there is any chemistry. Trust your instincts.

- Tell a friend when and where you are going, and that it is an internet meeting. Have them call you at a predetermined time.

- Choose a well-lit, open, crowded public place, such as a coffee shop.

- Daytime is best, lighting is good. Wear business attire or a conservative outfit.

- Keep the conversation light, no personal information (job, school, home).

- The meeting is dutch. Pay your own bill quickly with cash and without hesitation.

- Further disclosure if there is mutual interest. Give your real name and consider showing each other ID or DL, but cover critical info (DOB, home address, DL number). Take a photo of them with your camera phone. Tell them you will talk soon on the phone.

- Run a background check. They are available online and relatively cheap (www. peoplefinders.com).

- Remember that anyone can act nice for ten minutes. You still do not know them.

First Date

- Do not have them pick you up at home. Drive yourself.

- Do not drink alcohol, but if you must, be vigilant (See DFSA).

- Let a friend know who you are out with, where you are going, and when you will be back. Prearrange a safety call.

- Call someone while you are out: friend, family, brother or buddy. Women: Invent a big brother if you do not have one.

- These precautions are not just for women. Men are victims of theft, scams, assault, and rape by women, women with male accomplices using them as lures, and by men. Be smart.

Fire

There are 1.6 million fires in the US every year, one every 19 seconds.

Every dwelling should have fire extinguishers, smoke detectors and carbon monoxide detectors. These are cheap and readily available. Learn how to check them and keep them fully functional.

Fires destroy property which can be replaced, and take lives which cannot. Preparation saves lives. House fires spread with surprising ferocity. You have to act fast. Humans die at 212°F and heat can exceed 1100°F in the fire and 300° in the rest of the house. Smoke creates complete darkness, and will burn your lungs when inhaled. All this happens within three minutes. Every second counts.

Smoke Alarms

Smoke alarms detect fire by sensing airborne particles. They are inexpensive, easy to install, and priceless. To save lives, they must be used properly:

• There are two sensing technologies: Ionization and Photoelectric. Each has advantages, so experts recommend using dual technology units.

• Install a unit on each floor, hallway and bedroom.

• Follow manual for testing, cleaning and replacing batteries. Use the best batteries available.

• These alarms are working constantly, and will eventually wear out. The technology advances as well. Replace them every 10 years.

Carbon Monoxide Alarms

Carbon monoxide is a tasteless, invisible, odorless gas produced by household appliances. It is a leading cause of accidental poisoning in the US and a silent killer. Your only protection is an alarm, and one should be added to the smoke alarms to complete your fire protection package. Change every five years as they wear out and the technology advances.

The Escape Plan

Prepare an escape plan. Realize that evacuation should take less than two minutes. The house will be thick with smoke, and fumes will make you sick and weak. A well drilled escape plan can save lives:

• Learn two ways out of each room.

- Have an exit plan from any second floor (fire ladder).

- Establish a meeting place so everyone can be counted.

- Practice and drill until perfect.

Fire in a Building

- Call 911 and pull alarm if you smell smoke or see fire.

- Leave the building immediately.

- Leave your valuables behind.

- Always use stairs or emergency exits. <u>Never use an elevator</u>.

- <u>Stay low and go</u>. Cover your mouth and nose with a wet cloth.

- Crawl under the smoke. Smoke inhalation kills by heat, fumes, asphyxia and toxins.

- Feel closed doors with the back of your hand for superheated doorknob or door. If it is hot, there is fire on the other side. Choose another door.

- If you catch fire…<u>STOP, DROP and ROLL</u> until the fire goes out.

- If you are trapped in a room, put clothes or tape around the doors and vents to prevent smoke from entering the room. Call 911 and tell them where you are.

- Once you are out, do not go back in. Let the firefighters do their job.

- Talk to the firefighters if you know someone is still in the building and give details of their location.

Fire Extinguishers

Fire extinguishers are rated for different fires. There are specific units for different types of fires (combustibles/flammable liquids/electrical); you may need several. If you only have one extinguisher, choose an A-B-C rated unit. Go to www.kidde.com for more information and warnings about when to use.

To Use a Fire Extinguisher, Remember PALSS;

- **P**ull safety pin.

- **A**im **L**ow at base of fire.

- **S**queeze lever slowly.

- **S**weep side to side evenly until out.

Do <u>not</u> try to fight anything but small, contained early fires.
Do <u>not</u> play firefighter. The first priority is to evacuate everyone, then call 911.

Fire Prevention

Most house fires start in the kitchen. Keep a kitchen fire extinguisher nearby and learn how to fight kitchen fires correctly. Most fatalities are caused by smoking or candles. Develop a habit of fully extinguishing all materials and never smoke in bed.

- Kitchen Fire – Rehearse and drill your escape plan. Have a phone and extinguisher accessible <u>away</u> from likely source of fire. Small fires in pans or oven can be contained by placing lid on pan (protect yourself with oven mitt) or by closing oven door. Do <u>not</u> try to carry to sink for dousing. For larger fire, use extinguisher rated: 10-B: C. If no extinguisher, use a fire blanket or baking soda. Do not throw water on grease fires (will spread the fire or backsplash and burn you) or electrical fires (will electrocute you).

- Home Fire – Rehearse and drill. Prevention is key: Keep flammables away from heat, limit candles, etc. <u>www.homesafetycouncil.org</u>. When a fire breaks out: <u>Evacuate everyone then call 911</u>. If the fire is small and contained, use extinguisher 3-A:40-B:C, being sure that you have a clear escape path and rooms are not filled with smoke.

- Vehicle Fire – Common, dangerous and deadly due to gas, oil, flammable fluids and plastics. The vast majority of vehicle fires are caused by mechanical/electrical malfunctions, not accidents. Frequently visually inspect your car's engine and wiring; check for fluid leaks, frayed wires, cracked hoses. Smoke, backfires and odors are danger signs. Have your vehicle inspected annually by a professional mechanic.

Vehicle Fires

Stop safely off the road, turn off ignition and put in *Park* and set brake. Get out of car and move 100 feet away from vehicle in case it explodes. Call 911. Do <u>not</u> go back to car.

Dog Bites

In the US, 4.5 million people are bitten by dogs every year, almost a million require medical treatment and tens of thousands need extensive surgery. Criminal and civil penalties for pet attacks are increasing, with zero tolerance for irresponsible owners. If you own a pet, beware of the dangers and consequences if it attacks someone. Your homeowners insurance may not cover you. Legal costs can be financially catastrophic and your pet will probably be quarantined and destroyed.

To Help Prevent Dog Bites:

• Never pet, hug, approach or bend your face toward a strange dog.

• Stay out of lunging reach of any dog, even if leashed.

• Avoid eye contact with the dog.

• Never approach dogs while they are eating, sleeping, sick or with their puppies.

• Never try to separate fighting animals.

• Never leave a young child alone with any pet.

• Remember, animals react unpredictably and with blinding speed.

• In the event of any animal bite, seek medical attention.

If you own a pet, consider the following to minimize the risk it will attack:

• Keep your pet on a leash and under control when entertaining houseguests, and always on a leash in public. Remember, an animal can lunge 3 feet. Keep leash taut.

• Do not take pets into malls, stores, grocery stores, restaurants.

• Spay or neuter your pet. This significantly reduces aggression and risk of biting.

• Never play aggressive games (tug of war, wrestling, riding) with dogs.

• Socialize your pet. Teach it to interact well with humans.

Firearm Safety

Firearms are second only to motor vehicles in causing death, injury and disability in the US and firearms are the second leading cause of death in people ages 10-24. There are approximately 30,000 firearm related deaths by murder or suicide and over 200,000 nonfatal gunshot wounds yearly. With over 300 million firearms in the US, an understanding of basic firearm handling and safety is critical. Take an NRA gun safety or hunting safety class to learn the basics, even if you never intend to hunt, own or use a firearm.

There Are No Accidental Shootings

There is no such thing as an accidental shooting or accidental discharge of a firearm. Modern firearms have solid, often multiple safety mechanisms, internal and external. Shootings are the result of operator error or negligence, improper weapon handling or lack of knowledge about a specific weapon. Learn and practice firearm safety.

The Five Cardinal Rules of Firearm Safety

<u>Every Gun Is Always Loaded</u> – No matter what someone tells you, or even if you personally checked it two hours ago…no matter what, always treat every gun as if it were loaded.

<u>Never Point The Gun At Anything You Are Not Willing To Destroy</u> – Keeping the muzzle pointed in a safe direction is absolutely critical, and requires constant attention and thought. Safe is <u>not</u>: up in the air, at a hard concrete surface, at a neighbor's wall. A modern high velocity round can travel miles, through masonry and drywall, and still kill.

<u>Keep Your Finger Off The Trigger Until You Are Ready To Fire</u> – Keep the finger out of the trigger guard, preferably on the side of the frame or body of the weapon, until absolutely ready to fire, and until the weapon is on target.

<u>Know Your Target And What Is Behind It</u> – Bullets can travel through your target. And if you miss, where will the bullet go? Will it strike someone or something else? You are responsible.

<u>Always Maintain Control of Your Weapon And Know How to Use It</u> – This is paramount to your safety, and the safety of others who may encounter the weapon, unintended by you. You are responsible.

Assert Your Rights

When you encounter a firearm, demand that all the safety rules be followed. Never assume anyone knows or will follow safety rules.

Your life is on the line.

Additional Rules

- Never use alcohol, drugs or OTC drugs when shooting. These impair body functions and judgment.

- Always immediately inspect, visually and with a finger, to be sure no round is in the chamber.

- A weapon is only safe if empty of ammunition and the chamber is open.

- Never trust the safety or assume that safety mechanism is working.

- Always use approved eye protection (clear or amber lens, high impact, wraparound).

- Always use approved ear protection; earplugs + earmuffs are the best.

- Never assume that others, even those with a military or law enforcement background, are knowledgeable or safe. Range accidents occasionally occur even with highly trained professionals.[9]

- Take control of situations involving firearms. There is no second chance.

- Worn old surplus weapons can be dangerous, explode when fired with modern high pressure ammunition, or have an inoperable safety.

- Be aware of the ejection path on semiautomatic weapons.

- Be aware of side blast, back blast and collateral forces on weapons.

- Only use safe and correct, commercially made ammunition. Do not use old, military surplus or hand loads.

- Bullets can travel easily through drywall, wood, even concrete, and kill innocent people in the next apartment, house or car. Never fire a weapon into the air. The bullet will come down and can kill.

- After shooting, be sure all weapons are empty with the safety on or broken down, and properly stored away from ammunition.

- Clean up after shooting. You will be covered in powder residue and lead dust and bullet shavings. Lead is highly toxic, and remains in the body forever, causing brain

---

9 Personal communication, Rangemaster, Usery Mountain Shooting Range. Feb 2010.

damage and birth defects. Thoroughly wash your hands and face, blow your nose and rinse your mouth. Shower and launder your clothes.

- Do not shoot in indoor ranges that are not well ventilated. Lead dust and shavings are toxic.

- Visit a local gun shop and take the opportunity to see different weapons, handle them, cycle them, learn them so that you know the basics of how a revolver, semiautomatic pistol, shotgun and rifle function. Learn the difference between single action and double action, pump and automatic, bolt action and semiautomatic design. Learn the positions and functions of safety mechanisms on weapons. Learn to load and unload a variety of weapons (you will not be allowed to do this in a gun store for safety reasons, but you can learn the procedure).

- If there is a firearm in the home, everyone, <u>adults and children</u>, must learn the basic safety rules in dealing with a firearm. Your life or another's depends on it.

Potentially Lethal Weapon Malfunctions

<u>Squib</u>: This occurs when the cartridge ignites and fires, but with reduced power. The cause is usually the powder; the recoil and/or report of the gunshot may be weak. The danger is that the bullet is still lodged in the barrel, plugging it. If another round is fired, the gun will catastrophically explode causing death or serious injury. In the event of a squib, keep the weapon pointed in a safe direction, immediately safe the weapon and examine the barrel to be sure it is clear. Have the weapon evaluated by an expert before resuming firing.

<u>Hangfire</u>: This occurs when the firing pin strikes but the round does not ignite immediately. This may be caused by a faulty firing pin or more commonly by a faulty primer, improperly stored ammunition, old or poor quality ammunition. A hangfire may explode at any time; in other words, the primer or powder charge may be slow burning and ignite a while <u>after</u> the firing pin struck, either in the weapon or in your hand. This can be fatal. In the event of a hangfire, keep weapon aimed in a safe direction as it could go off at any time, wait <u>2 minutes</u>, then remove magazine and unload the cartridge and dispose of properly. Inspect the barrel for obstruction. Have the weapon evaluated by an expert before firing.

Water Safety

Ten Americans drown every day. Many more receive long-term brain damage from near drowning incidents. Most adult drownings occur in open water (rivers/lakes/ocean) because we are used to swimming pools, and are unprepared for the dangers of tides, currents, undertows and open water. Humans are not well adapted for water: Olympic swimmers, in sprint distances, swim 4 mph. Distance swimmers are slower. A typical gentle tidal flow of just 5 mph will exhaust and drown even an Olympic swimmer in his prime.

Open Water Safety

- When arriving at a beach for the first time, spend time watching the water, currents, waves. Ask the locals about conditions and the underwater topography. Be careful.

- Tides are cyclic, twice daily movements of water on and off shore, massive loads of water that are irresistible forces to respect and fear.

- Currents are streams of water within the ocean, sometimes constant, sometimes fluctuating, and always dangerous. Especially dangerous around cuts between land and underwater geography like shoals, sandbars or reefs. Typically, they are found in areas of great interest to divers, swimmers and boaters.

- Riptides are not tides, but narrow, fast currents that take water back out into the ocean from the beach. If caught in a rip current, do not swim against the rip current and do not panic. Do not try to swim back to shore. Swim parallel to the shore until out of the current's grip, and then swim to shore. If you tire: Relax, float out until the current fades and then swim parallel to shore until away from rip, and then swim in. Remember: If you keep your head, you can easily survive. Panic kills.

- Check weather forecasts before swimming or boating.

- Always swim or dive with the buddy system. And that means keep a close and frequent watch on your buddy. Things happen fast.

- Never mix alcohol with swimming or boating. Half of serious injuries involve drugs or alcohol.

- Swim near a lifeguard and know your flags: Green/Favorable, Yellow/Caution, Red/Danger, Two Red Flags/Beach Closed.

- Use surfboards, boogie boards, anything buoyant to make swimming easier.

- When boating use USCG flotation devices. Be aware of the danger of the propeller when in the water. Do not drink and drive a boat.

- Never dive into pools, lakes or rivers. Never dive where you cannot see the bottom. Unseen obstructions, trees or rocks cause spinal injuries and drowning.

- Learn CPR. Encourage your buddy to learn CPR.

Kitchen Safety

There are 76 million cases of food poisoning every year. Additionally, many accidents and household fires occur in the kitchen, making kitchen safety a high priority.

Shark Glove

Purchase a Normark Rapala Fillet glove made of a cut resistant fabric. This glove may save a trip to the ER. And <u>never</u> try to cut anything frozen.

- Refrigerator – Keep at 40°F. Put cooked food immediately in the refrigerator. If left out for more than 2 hours, discard. Discard refrigerated food/leftovers after 3-5 days. Thaw foods in the refrigerator, not on the counter. If power outage occurs, do not open door, food should stay good for 24 hours. Discard any questionable food. Never refreeze thawed food.

- Microwave – Use <u>microwave safe</u> containers only. Others can leach chemicals into your food. Use only lead free ceramic mugs/bowls. Use caution. See Superheating.

- Stove – Use new, high temperature oven mitts and pads to handle pots. Keep handles of pots and pans safe; not over burners or sticking out from stove for toddler to pull down on or someone to bump. Never leave anything on the stove unattended.

Microwave Safety and Superheating

Microwave ovens simplify daily life, and save energy and time. While they are in many ways safer than conventional ovens, they have dangers. Microwave ovens have a magnetron that emits electromagnetic energy, which strikes the water molecules within the food, heating it from the outside in.

Potential Hazards

• Radiation – The FDA has done extensive testing of microwave ovens, and has established standards for leakage. The risk of injury by radiation is very small, and decreases rapidly as you move away from the microwave. However, you should never operate microwaves with poor, worn or damaged doors, hinges, latches or seals. Never operate a microwave if the door does not close and latch securely. Do not stand too close to the microwave or peer inside when it is operating.

• Superheating – This occurs when water or liquid is overheated, often in a new, smooth cup or for too long. The liquid enters a superheated state, at a temperature above boiling, but remains still and calm with no bubbles. Then, when the cup is moved or if something is mixed into it, the liquid will burst into a boil and explode out of the vessel, burning or scalding face and hands. Reduce risk: Read manual for cook time and power for liquids and never overheat liquid or repeatedly reheat liquid. Use old scratched cups. Mix in sugar, salt, or coffee before heating. Insert wooden stir stick in liquid prior to heating. After heating, tap cup with wooden spoon before touching. Always keep face and hands away from open door and container; cautiously test. NOTE: These precautions should reduce risk, but hot liquid always has potential to injure, and caution must always be used, especially when feeding/serving infants and children.

• Fire – Metal reflects microwave energy, causing sparks or fire. Never put metal, aluminum foil, cutlery, or glasses/plates/etc. with precious metal leaf inlays or appliqués in microwave. Clean the microwave per manual; never use steel wool or scouring pads. Do not operate the microwave empty as this can damage the magnetron or cause fire.

• Hot spots and cool containers – Microwaves heat food, not containers. Often the cup or dish will be cool, but the food very hot, leading to misjudgment and burns. Stir food thoroughly to mix hot spots. Use extreme care with baby food and children. Never heat food in a sealed container; trapped steam may scald when opened.

Read the owner's manual thoroughly, as each microwave is different.

193

Food Preparation

- Fresh Foods – Vegetables, fruits, and produce should be washed thoroughly with a brush and tap water, and rinsed to remove wax, pesticides and dirt. This is especially true for anything grown on or contacting the ground, or of foreign origin. Sanitary conditions aren't always used in fertilizing or harvesting these products.

- Eggs – Never eat anything with raw eggs. Salmonella can live <u>inside</u> the shell, and is a major cause of illness. Cook eggs thoroughly.

- Meat – *E.coli* on beef and salmonella on chicken cause illness and occasionally death. Refrigerate fresh meat/poultry for 1-2 days max. Clean and prep meat and then thoroughly clean prep area with warm soap, water and bleach solution. Run cutting board through dishwasher. Consider having two cutting boards, one just for meats and one for fresh, uncooked foods. Always discard marinades after use. Always cook meats using a meat thermometer; looks are deceiving.

- Cutting Boards – Consider purchasing synthetic cutting boards; wooden boards harbor bacteria, are hard to clean, and warp in the dishwasher.

- Seafood – Use great caution in buying seafood. Purchase only from reputable sources with high turnover. Check the packaging and freshness. Fresh fish will smell like the sea, not smell "fishy".

- Disinfect – Keep a bleach solution (1 teaspoon bleach/1quart water) for sanitizing cutting boards, countertops, sinks and drains. Use often. Clean as you go. Clean tops of drink/soup cans and all canned food before opening to remove warehouse grime. Clean sponges and scrub brushes frequently in the dishwasher.

Produce Handling and Produce Safety

Bacteria, viruses, pesticides, contaminants and irrigation waste get on produce where it is grown, harvested or packed. They may cause food borne illness (diarrhea, nausea, vomiting, stomach ache, flu like symptoms) or death. This is especially true in third world countries where raw sewage (night soil) is used as fertilizer.

Prevention

- Do not purchase bruised fruit.

- Avoid fresh cut produce, such as a half of melon or sliced fruit.

- Do not eat raw sprouts because rinsing will not remove bacteria.

- Separate produce from meat, fish and poultry in the refrigerator.

- Keep meat products from contaminating your produce when cooking.

- Refrigerate perishable and pre-cut produce at 40° F or below. Ask your grocer what is perishable.

- Wash your hands for 20 seconds with warm water and soap prior to all food preparation.

- Wash all produce thoroughly with water only (soap or detergent is not recommended by the FDA) before eating or preparing. This includes produce that has a peel.

- Use a scrub brush on melons and hard surface fruit. Melons grow on the ground and can have dirt and bacteria that are carried into the inner fruit when sliced.

- Drying with cloth or paper towel will further reduce bacteria.

- Cut away bruises or damaged areas.

- Wash cutting boards, counters and utensils with soap and water or bleach after preparing foods, especially meats, fish and poultry. Use sanitizers with bleach or one teaspoon of bleach in one quart of water to wash countertops and cutting surfaces.

Pearls

- Choose produce from the USA because health standards are more consistent.

- Check country of origin on all food you buy: produce, canned, frozen.

- Be especially careful if your immune system is weakened or if you are feeding young children.

- Buy only pasteurized fruit juice.

Dishwashers

A dishwasher (DW) is essential for a healthy sanitary kitchen. Clean dishes improve the flavor and presentation of your food, and reduce food borne diseases. To maximize the efficiency of this appliance, it helps to understand its magical inner workings.

Function - The cycle starts as hot water submerges the heating element in the bottom tub recess, then is heated to scalding (home units sanitize at ~150°, but do not sterilize), mixed with the prewash dose of detergent and pumped through the spray arm at high pressure to jet clean the dishes. Enzymes loosen and digest baked on food and a macerator liquefies food particles and pumps the effluent out to the drain or garbage disposal. More soap is added during the main wash cycle, and then the clean dishes are thoroughly rinsed and heated until dry.

Detergents – Use only products specifically formulated for a DW. Powders dissolve better than gels; they have additives to reduce spots, soften water and maintain performance. Avoid cheap powders as they cause damage. Enzymes and green biodegradable detergents clean without using polluting phosphates. Rinse aids are recommended to speed drying and reduce spots.

Loading and Unloading - The quality of cleaning depends on the quality of loading. Jets must hit evenly, and have access to all recesses of the dishes and utensils. Load upper rack with any plastic items to avoid melting, and place the dirtiest items directly over the jets. Place utensils in the silverware bins loosely, handles up and eating surface down, no spooning or nesting. Always load knives and sharp items point down. Unload with clean hands, not touching eating surface of utensils and dishes.

Enhancing Dishwasher Performance and Efficiency - Do not rinse and hand wash dishes before loading; this is unnecessary and simply wastes time and ~6500 gal water per year. Just scrape large scraps and bones into the trash and load. Never put anything unsuitable (paint brushes, car parts, rugs, antiques, hats, etc.) in as these can damage or contaminate the DW. No nonstick pans, lead crystal, gold, pewter, brass, tin, bronze, disposable plastic or aluminum utensils or plates. Make sure your kitchen items are DW safe before loading them. Run the tap until water is hot, then start cycle. Use the shorter cycle (80-100 min) to save water and energy. Read your manual as some models have a filter to clean.

Maintenance - Check the spray arms for free, easy motion and that the jets are unobstructed and clean. Be sure the detergent cup opens and releases the soap properly; clean it regularly; some models have dual cups. Check the heating element recess for debris and lost silverware. Lastly, periodically check the door, door latch, sink vent, filter and hoses.

Laundry

Laundry is about far more than just dirt. Properly laundering your clothes, towels and bedding significantly reduces unwanted bacteria, viruses, fungi, dust mites and other unhealthy contaminants. Perhaps equally important, clean, fresh clothing has a huge impact on your appearance and personal hygiene. Clothing, especially shirts, underwear and socks, should only be worn once, and then laundered. You cannot detect your own body odor.

The Basics

Detergent types: Powders are best for mud, dirt, clay. Liquid is best for grease, oil, food stains. For delicate or handwash cycles use Ivory Snow® or Woolite® which are formulated specifically for gentle cycles. Use the recommended amount of detergent; too much leaves soapy residue on clothes, too little leaves dirt. Buy only laundry detergent labeled hypoallergenic and unscented as it will have minimal additives. Additives can cause allergic itching and dermatitis, as well as disrupt sleep significantly (from bedding, sheets, pajamas). Fragrances conflict with your cologne or perfume.

Bleach is necessary to sanitize and brighten <u>whites</u>. Do not use on colors.

Fabric Softener can permanently stain fabrics if undiluted and has fragrance that can conflict with cologne and perfume. An unscented, hypoallergenic fabric softener is the best choice.

Laundry Time

Read the care labels on your clothing before you purchase them. Some items may only be dry cleaned, others require special handling.

- Sort and wash by color: Light/medium/dark colors, whites alone with bleach.

- New garments or fabrics (jeans, dark sheets or towels) should be washed alone, as dye frequently bleeds heavily in first and second washings.

- Heavily soiled clothes should be washed separately (heavily soiled work garments or sweaty gym clothes).

- Lingerie should be done alone, in a single load, using lingerie bag.

- Pretreat or prewash as needed. www.clothesline.com.

- Sort by cycle: Separate clothes by fabric type and the cycle you will run: Whites/ Colors/Permanent Press/Delicates. Modern washers have computerized custom cycles for each type of fabric, and correct use will significantly improve both cleaning and prolong the lifetime of the garment. Within each cycle choice, there are usually settings for heavy, medium or light soiling. Use the appropriate setting to save energy and the fabric.

• Whites: Add bleach to bleach dispenser to minimize risk of damage to fabric and assure mixing at the right time. If no dispenser, add to water after 5-10 minutes of the wash cycle to maximize results. Use ¾ cup for regular and 1 ¼ cups for large load.

• Water T° for Wash cycle: HOT for whites, bedding, sheets, pillowcases, towels and sturdy colorfast fabrics. WARM for permanent press, colorfast, synthetic, moderate soiled fabrics. COLD for lightly soiled, dark colors, bright colors, permanent press, synthetics. Cold is the safest for the fabric and the environment.

• Water T° for Rinse cycle: Always use COLD.

• Immediately remove clothes from washer at end of cycle.

• Dryer: Use appropriate setting. Regular for cottons; Permanent Press for most or all synthetics, knits, dress shirts and pants; Delicate for lingerie and lightweight performance synthetics like Under Armour®, Dri-Fit® or Coolmax®.

• Remove knits/jerseys/heavy fabrics while slightly damp and hang on padded fabric hangers to decrease wrinkling.

• Ironing: If necessary, iron items while damp at correct iron setting. Use the spray mister in the iron or a spray bottle to wet fabric before ironing. Always fill the iron with distilled water, and empty the iron of water after use to prevent rust and mineral buildup.

MOTOR VEHICLE SAFETY

"Better a thousand times careful than once dead."

Proverb

Pearls

General

- Never drink and drive.

- Never text or talk on the phone in the car. Studies show this is as bad as being drunk.

- Always wear seat belts and shoulder harnesses. Properly. No exceptions.

- Adjust the seat, mirrors and belts to fit you perfectly.

- Always drive with running lights on in daylight.

- Adjust all three mirrors correctly. There are tutorials and techniques to adjust your mirrors for maximum view (www.cartalk.com and www.caranddriver.com). Know what's behind you and in other lanes, especially when changing lanes.

- Use your blinkers. Don't do it for the other driver; do it for your own safety. Let everyone know where you're going. They are less likely to hit you.

- Drive the speed limit: better mpg, less fatalities, less severe injuries. Allow extra time for all your trips so you are not in a hurry.

- Sleeping at the wheel causes 100,000 car accidents a year. If you are drowsy, your judgment is impaired the equivalent to 5 drinks. Do not drive when tired.

- Practice defensive driving. Focus on the road. Most accidents can be prevented with defensive driving.

- Eliminate internal distractions: phones, music, texting, multiple friends talking, makeup, pets on lap, etc.

- Pets in car: Dogs and cats do not really understand vehicular travel. Nor are they protected by seat belts in the event of accident. Keep pets in a travel cage to protect them and yourself.

- Never hitchhike or pick up hitchhikers.

- Driving in the rain: The first 15 minutes are the most dangerous, as rain lifts oil and grease making the road very slick until more rain washes it clean. Drive slowly.

- Never smoke when filling your car with gasoline. *Flames + gas = fire.*

- Maintain a fuel level of ¼ or more at all times. Running out of gas is difficult and can put you at unnecessary risk.

- Do not fill your car's gas tank when a gasoline tanker is filling the tanks of the station. The high speed and volume of gas entering the station's gas holding tanks stirs up sediment that normally is at the bottom of the tank. Filling your car with this gasoline can clog fuel filter or damage the engine.

Old ER Dictum:

Nothing good ever happens after midnight. Stay off the roads after midnight, because the drunks are driving home and even the sober are tired and weary.

Intersections

- Beware - Left turns across traffic are inherently dangerous.

- Always look right and left at intersections, especially when light changes. Red light runners kill.

- Never turn wheels while waiting to turn across traffic. If you are rear ended, you will be thrust forward and turned into oncoming traffic.

- Do not swing out wide for turns. This is totally unnecessary unless you are pulling a rig.

The Three Second Rule

One of the most important defensive driving techniques is maintaining a proper cushion of time and space between your vehicle and the vehicles around you. One method is to keep one vehicle length per 10 mph between you and the vehicle in front of you. A more precise method is to allow a 3 second interval between cars for daylight, good driving conditions, and 6 seconds for nighttime or wet, poor driving conditions. In heavy rain or snow, increase to a 9 second cushion because both human reaction times and vehicle response times are longer.

Learn the method, and remember that the faster you drive, the greater the 3 second distance will become. Practice in daylight, in excellent conditions, until it becomes second nature. As you are driving, notice when the car in front of you passes by a sign, or bridge, or clear landmark. Never taking your eyes off the road or losing concentration, begin counting "one-one thousand-two-one thousand-three-one thousand". You should pass the landmark at 3 seconds. Once you get a feel for that distance, you will no longer need to constantly divert your attention in counting.

For more information, see www.smartmotorist.com.

Highway Driving

- Use the 3/6/9 second rule to maintain a safe distance between you and car ahead of you. Do not get boxed in by traffic. If someone is tailgating you, allow them by. Always leave yourself an escape path.

- Always check your blind spot when changing lanes.

- While driving on the highway, look at your escape routes (median strip, shoulder, adjoining lanes). Never get into a position in traffic where you have no escape path to avoid a collision.

- Be especially careful where highways split and at major turnoffs. Surprised drivers make rash, last minute lane changes without thinking and can cause serious accidents.

- Do not pass on bridges. When passing another vehicle you need an emergency escape route. A bridge or any other obstruction does not allow lateral movement.

- Do not stay in another vehicle's blind spot. Move through or maintain a position behind the blind spot.

- If you have engine trouble or a flat tire (with no Fix-a-Flat available) and your cell phone does not have a signal, drive on a poorly functioning engine or tire until you are in cell range (look for a hill). Always consider your personal safety and get help first; any damage to your car can be repaired.

Maintenance

- Join the American Automobile Association (AAA). Among the many benefits of AAA (discounts, travel service, maps), the most important is reliable and reputable roadside service for flat tires, breakdowns or other emergencies. Put the AAA emergency number in your cell phone. When you call the AAA, notify them if you are in a dangerous traffic area, and they will make you a priority.

- Find a reputable garage for your routine maintenance and emergency car care. Do this before you have to have your vehicle towed. Realize that there are many proprietary parts/electronics in modern vehicles. Often dealerships are the best choice.

- Check your car before any long trip. Oil level, water level, tire pressure, lug nuts, brakes, fuel, emergency kit, food and water.

Car Emergency Kit

Accidents happen fast. You will be dazed, rattled or even injured. Prepare yourself with a full kit.

- License and Registration.
- In glove box: Insurance documents, agent's number, insurance company 800 number, family contacts, 3 redacted copies of insurance card (no home address or liability limit info) for police and other driver.
- AAA roadside emergency card.
- Disposable 35mm camera with flash or camera on your cell phone.
- Small paper journal and pen.
- Cell phone and 12V charger.
- Fire extinguisher, small, 1A10BC or 2A10BC.
- Flashlight LED powerful Surefire G2/Energizer Swivel standup, spare batteries and bulb.
- Multi-tool – Leatherman® or Gerber®.
- Spare headlight bulbs – know how to replace.
- Safety goggles, work gloves, rags, towels, Windex®.
- Windshield washer fluid.
- Tire pressure gauge, tire tread depth gauge.
- 2 cans Fix-A-Flat®.
- Jack and lug wrench – know their location.
- Wheel chock.
- Assortment of spare fuses – know fuse box site.
- Water, powdered sports drink and energy bars.
- Reflective emergency space blanket.
- White cloth emergency distress flag.
- Jumper cables, heavy gauge, 20+ feet.
- PortaJump® battery booster.
- First aid kit.
- Road reflectors (flares are highly flammable).

- Light sticks and waterproof matches.
- $20 small bills emergency cash.

Additional items for a long distance road trip:

- Basic tools: screwdrivers/sockets/wrenches.
- Coolant hose repair kit and hose clamps.
- One day's food/water per person.
- GPS
- CB radio or satellite phone service – Vital when no cell service reaches.

Additional items for winter driving:

- Windshield scraper.
- Snow chains, grip treads and tow strap. Learn in advance how these are used correctly.
- Blankets, hand warmers, warm clothes.
- Shovel – military folding shovel for snow.
- Bag of cat litter – cheap instant traction.

Basic Automobile Safety

Automobile accidents obey the laws of physics. While there is no way to avoid all accidents, there are things you can do to minimize risk and increase your protection should a collision occur.

Mass:

The heavier your vehicle is, the safer you are.

Visibility 1:

Your ability to see outwards: window size, mirrors, vehicle design.

The more you can see, the better.

Visibility 2:

How easily and quickly your vehicle is seen by other drivers depends on paint color, running lights, size. The more visible you are, the better.

Maintenance:

Tires, brakes, lights, seatbelts, airbags etc. must function well.

Inherent Vehicle Safety:

Research vehicle safety with consumerreports.org and safercar.gov

Motor Vehicle Accidents (MVAs)

There are more than 6 million auto accidents yearly, resulting in 34,000 deaths. The highest fatality rate occurs on Friday and Saturday night between 9 PM and 3 AM. MVAs are a leading cause of death and long term disability and the financial cost is estimated at over $200 billion. It is an epidemic.

Understand that getting in your car constitutes the greatest risk of death or injury you face as an adult. It is not a right to be taken lightly. Failure to respect safe, sane, responsible driving laws can have tragic and irreversible results: financial loss in excess of insurance coverage, lost wages, loss of driver's license, civil liability and damages, criminal charges, imprisonment (mandatory for DUI), physical injury, disability and death. Avoid accidents at all cost, but know what to do when one occurs.

Causes of MVAs

The major causes of MVAs are fatigue, distractions, alcohol or drug use, and cell phone use. All are preventable.

Prepare Before Accident

- Car Emergency Kit

- Insurance agent name and number. Review your policy re: authorized repair shops, car rentals, towing and other details. Dealerships are often preferred. Pick the best.

- Prepare several copies of a censored insurance card to be given to police and other driver. To other drivers you are only required to provide: insurance company, policy number, your name and means of contact (cell). Do not show home address, phone, work info or liability limits and policy info to avoid stalking and discourage lawsuits.

- Cell phone with three emergency contacts including your insurance carrier phone number already entered.

- Disposable 35mm camera or cell phone with camera

- First aid kit

After the Accident

- Stop and remain in the car. Do not leave scene of accident.

- Immediately establish your personal safety, check yourself for injury and assess the situation.

- Call 911 to report the accident and any injuries, then call your insurance company, and finally your friends or family.

- Relax. At this point, if you are not injured, you are just collecting data and exchanging information.

- Never say "sorry" or suggest in any way that the accident is your fault even if you think it might be. You do not know the law or if the other driver is impaired. Let law enforcement investigate and make that assessment.

- Photograph the accident site and both vehicles from every possible angle before moving cars. Write in your journal your recollection of the crash.

- Check local and state laws re: moving a vehicle after an accident. If the car is creating a safety hazard or you are concerned for your personal safety, move the car to a safer area. Take a photo first, if possible.

- Do not argue, accuse or fight with other driver.

- Airbags can spontaneously deploy <u>after</u> an accident. Do not sit in car until airbag is checked and safe.

- Do not disclose the financial limits of your insurance.

- Obtain license number, type of car, driver's name, cell phone number and insurance information. Give the other driver the same information and nothing more (no addresses, home phone number, place of work)

- Get the passenger's name, any injuries, policy and phone numbers.

- Get names of witnesses, their license numbers or vehicle descriptions.

- Write down what happened while everything is fresh in your mind.

- Talk with the police in a calm and respectful manner. Do not argue with anyone.

- Can you drive the car? Ask the police and insurance company. If vehicle is disabled, have them arrange towing to an authorized repair shop.

- Remain calm. If you have any injuries, go to the hospital or call your doctor immediately.

Vehicle Breakdown

Safe Procedure

- Turn on your hazard lights/emergency flasher immediately, as soon as you notice a problem, even while you are still in traffic.

- Pull off the road as far as possible. The greatest danger in vehicle breakdown is being hit by a passing vehicle or causing an accident.

- If you are alone, be aware of your personal safety.

- Call 911, AAA and a family/friend to give your location and problem.

- Put a white handkerchief or cloth on the antenna and/or raise your hood.

- If you have a flare or safety triangle, place behind your parked car.

- Remain in your car with the doors locked if this is safe.

- If you have to get out of the car, exit on the passenger's side and stand to the other side of the guard rail, away from traffic.

- If someone stops and approaches your vehicle, talk through a cracked window. Ask them to call 911/Police for assistance or tell them you have already called 911/Police and everything is taken care of. Do not get in their car under any circumstances.

How to Fix a Flat Tire

Most every driver will have a flat tire during their lifetime. They are easy to fix and with the new tire sealant products available, effortless. If you have AAA, call them and they will come and fix your tire for you.

Prevention is simple: Check your tire pressure monthly. Every time you gas up, walk around the car and check tires for nails or damage.

- When you have a flat tire, your car may make a loud noise then slow down and become difficult to control.

- Pull over to a firm and safe part of the road, paved if possible. Turn on your emergency flashers or open hood. Place flares or reflective triangles at 10 foot intervals.

- Put the car in gear or *Park*. Apply parking brake.

- Inspect the damaged tire. If you have Fix-a-Flat®, follow instructions on bottle. Fix-a-Flat is an excellent but temporary fix. You will need to go to a tire or auto repair shop.

- If you do not have a tire sealant product, follow your auto manual's instructions to change the tire.

- Get all passengers, if any, out of the vehicle.

- Open trunk, remove jack, spare tire and wrench.

- Check spare tire pressure.

- Chock the diagonal wheel. This means block the diagonally opposite wheel from the flat tire with a heavy, immovable object to prevent the car from rolling forward off the jack. A commercial wheel chock is the best choice.

- Remove hubcap. Use wrench to loosen lug nuts on flat tire. When all nuts are just loose (but not off), place jack on flat surface in proper position outlined in your manual. Jack car up, remove lug nuts, remove tire and place on ground.

- Never get under car. Never rock car while on jack. Never allow anyone in the vehicle while it is up on the jack.

- Install spare and tighten lug nuts to contact. Lower car and firmly tighten lug nuts.

- Put flat tire and jack in trunk.

- Go to auto repair shop to have the tire repaired and vehicle inspected.

How to Jump Start a Car

Dead batteries are a common emergency, and can be dangerous. Over 6000 people suffer severe eye injuries yearly when car batteries filled with sulfuric acid and hydrogen gas explode. While everyone has jumper cables, most do not know how to use them correctly or safely.

Gear

Heavy gauge cables with strong spring clamps, heavy duty gloves and splash proof eye protection/goggles (Z-87).

Correct Method, Correct Order

Follow this sequence to jump a dead battery. Remember that many well intentioned "helpers" do not know the correct, safe technique to jump a battery. If you are unsure, call AAA, a tow service, or the police.

- Find a safe place to park the cars, away from traffic dangers. Turn off both ignitions and all accessories <u>except flashers</u>. Set parking brakes and put cars in *Park*. Read manual to see if jumping is permitted on your vehicle.

- No smoking, flames or sparks. Batteries explode.

- Use only heavy duty well insulated cables with good clamps. Red is positive (+) or hot. Black is (-) or ground.

- Keep the clamp ends of the cables separate at all times…just touching them for a millisecond can spark or short out.

- Clamp one red cable to the (+) pole of the dead battery.

- Clamp other red cable end to the (+) pole of the good battery.

- Clamp one black cable to the (-) pole of the good battery.

- Clamp the other black cable to a "ground" such as an unpainted metal surface on the engine block or frame of the car with the dead battery. In some new cars, there is a "ground" metal stud on the front of the engine block specifically for jump-starting cars. Do not attach to the dead battery, or any fuel lines, the carburetor injectors or moving parts. Be sure that the cable is clear of any fan blades, belts or other moving parts.

- Now, stand clear and start the good car. Idle for a few minutes

- Then start the car with the dead battery. Idle for a few minutes.

- Remove the cables in the REVERSE order, being very careful not to allow the clamps to touch each other, the vehicles' metal, or fall into the engine compartment.

211

- Drive the car cautiously, and do not turn it off until at an auto repair shop or safely home. Have the battery tested by a professional, and replaced or recharged as needed. Batteries have a 2-3 year life span, and damaged batteries should be replaced.

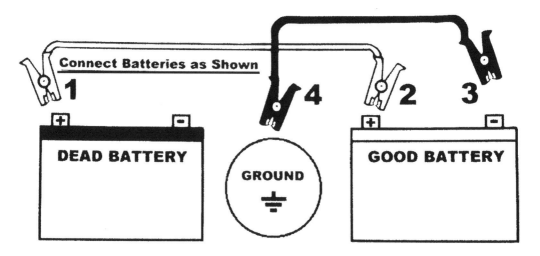

Diagram courtesy of Prevent Blindness America www.PreventBlindness.org

---

Summary of Sequence

RED-DEAD, RED-LIVE, BLACK-LIVE, BLACK-GROUND

- RED CABLE to the (+) pole of the DEAD battery.
- Other end of RED CABLE to the (+) pole of the LIVE battery.
- BLACK CABLE to the (-) pole of the LIVE battery.
- Other end of BLACK CABLE to "ground"

Talking to the Police

In your lifetime, you will have many interactions with authority: police, customs, security, military personnel. To serve and protect is a difficult profession. They deal with the worst of humanity and they deserve your sincere respect. Remember they need to assess you quickly and are trained to detect lies. Your behavior will influence the outcome. Bad attitude, bad outcome.

Know Your Rights

You are innocent until proven guilty. Furthermore, you have no requirement to prove your innocence. Remain quiet and do not divulge information. You can refuse a request to search your car. You can ask "Am I free to go?" Never run from the police, and never, ever touch an officer.

Traffic Stop

Traffic stops are extremely dangerous for police officers. Officer fatalities occur from ambush and being struck by other vehicles. There are no "routine traffic stops". Cooperate and hope for a warning.

When You See Flashing Lights Behind You:

- Slow down. Make sure he is after you.

- Pull over. Turn on flashers. If nighttime, turn on dome light.

- Roll your window down. Place your hands on the wheel at 10 and 2.

- Stay calm.

- Smile, be polite and courteous, and move slowly.

- Say "Yes, Officer?", then let him talk.

- Answer only the questions asked. Offer nothing extra. Keep it short and sweet.

- Do not argue or dispute. Do not lie. Say "I don't know."

- Accept the decision. There are legal options should you choose to contest at a later date.

Road Rage

Every year, 1500 injuries result from road rage. Understand that drivers who exhibit road rage are not rational and their behavior is unpredictable. When challenged they may react aggressively and escalate conflict on the road.

Prevention and Management

- Allow extra time for all trips, relax, and slow down.

- Be stress free when you drive. It will benefit you and others.

- Be courteous and think about the big picture. Help others get where they are going safely.

- Honk your horn <u>only</u> to warn someone of an impending danger, not to signal an error in their driving or your displeasure.

- Never tailgate. Maintain a safe distance. Allow other cars to merge.

- Use your signal when changing lanes or turning.

- Keep headlights at low beam.

- If someone cuts you off or merges in front of you, let them be. In the big picture, you will still get there, perhaps a second or two later.

- Never gesture or curse at another driver. People can read lips.

- Stay in the appropriate lane, never blocking the passing lane. If you are not moving with traffic get over to the slow lane, even if you are going the speed limit.

- Do not use your cell phone in the car. It is a distraction, and illegal in many states.

- Avoid eye contact or engaging an angry driver. The other driver may have just lost their job, be on medications/drugs, have psychiatric history or be armed. Avoid them at all costs.

- If harassed, lock your doors and windows. If in traffic, leave space for your vehicle to maneuver. Honk horn if someone is trying to break into your vehicle. Don't retaliate. Defuse, back off and slow down. Recall one of your own past stupid driving moves. We all have them.

- Never engage an angry driver. If they follow you, do not go home. Call 911 and go to a police station or public place.

- Your life is precious. Get there alive.

Motorcycles

Motorcycle fatalities have increased again this year, for the seventh year in a row. Speeding, alcohol and no formal training are causes. Most deaths are in age 20-29. Most accidents occur in first 500 miles of new bike or rider.

- Take the Motorcycle Safety Foundation Rider Course. <u>Never get on a bike without it</u>. <u>www.msf-usa.org</u>.

- Never ride on the back of any bike; the dynamics of bike handling change dramatically with a passenger loaded, and not all riders understand and can handle this. Not all passengers know how to move correctly.

- Always wear a helmet and Kevlar body armor.

- Be extremely cautious on a new bike. You will be unaccustomed to the power response, handling and balance, increasing risk of injury or death.

- Motorcycles are not a fashion accessory. They must be fitted to the rider's arm, leg and torso length. The wrong bike will increase your risk of injury.

- You may survive an automobile accident. It is very unlikely you will escape a motorcycle accident without injury, disfigurement, disability or worse.

- Remember, motorcycles are inherently unstable and riders are totally exposed. Automobiles often do not see the motorcyclist. Use every safety precaution and ride defensively.

Statistics prove that it is likely that you will have an accident on a motorcycle. Carry a card with hospital choice and name of personal physician on your body.

Basic Automobile Maintenance

Modern cars are extremely sophisticated, computerized engineering marvels that can last 200,000 miles if taken care of. Routine maintenance will prolong car life and prevent breakdowns in the middle of nowhere. Here are some things you should do:

- Read the manual and follow the maintenance schedule for your car.

- The Big Three: Tires, Lights, Wipers. All three of these wear out, and have a limited life span. ConsumersReports.org has excellent tire reviews for every climate and application. Lights, especially headlights, weaken. Consider replacement with new, high brightness halogen bulbs. Wipers should be changed at least yearly because they get brittle.

- On a monthly basis, check fluid levels (oil, transmission, radiator, brakes and window washing fluid).

- To check oil level, run car for 5 minutes before checking. Turn engine off and locate dipstick. Remove and wipe clean, then replace and remove. If oil is between the lines in the dipstick, it is good. If it is below, add a half quart and recheck. Do not overfill.

- Automatic transmission fluid level should be checked with the engine running. Find the dipstick, remove, wipe clean and replace. Remove and read. Unless there is a leak, the level should be normal.

- Radiator fluid level should be checked when the engine is *slightly* warm, not cold or hot. Read manual. The cooling system is pressurized and can burn you if hot. Never check radiator when the engine is on. The reservoir tank acts as both an overflow and storage tank for the radiator. Add fluid in a 50/50 mixture of coolant and water to the reservoir tank. If you have to open the radiator, place a towel over the cap when removing to protect yourself from hot splatter. Use caution.

- Brakes are a closed system and like the transmission fluid should not leak. Find the brake fluid reservoir and visually check level. If not at the line (usually 2/3 full), add the recommended fluid in the manual.

- Window washer fluid is usually housed in a clear reservoir that is labeled. Add water with Windex or premixed washer fluid from auto supply store. Be careful not to confuse this reservoir with the radiator reservoir.

- Change oil every 3-7500 miles (per manual). Use a quality oil filter.

- Change wiper blades every fall at minimum, twice a year in northern cold climates.

- Every 2-4 years, change: coolant, transmission fluid and all belts and hoses to avoid surprises.

- Use only recommended octane rating fuel.

- Rotate tires per schedule to increase mpg and decrease wear, usually 5-10,000 miles. Check your manual.

- Check tire pressure frequently. Recommended pressures are located inside driver side door frame. All tires leak. Low or high pressure is dangerous and decreases mpg, increases risk of rollover or catastrophic blowout.

- Tire quality and tread may be the most important safety issue of all. Check tire tread with thread gauge or quarter. Replace if less than 4/32" or if the top of the George Washington's head shows above tread. Tire tread is critical, especially in rain, snow or ice. If the tread is not deep enough, water, ice and snow cannot be channeled away and the tire will hydroplane with loss of control of the vehicle.

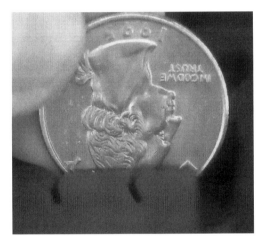 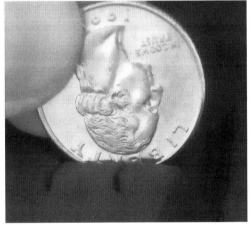

| Adequate tread | Replace this tire |

- Periodically check your emergency flasher.

- Clean the air filter regularly, especially in dusty areas. The engine has to breathe easily or your mpg will suffer.

- Have the brakes professionally inspected at any sign of trouble: fading, squealing, grinding, etc.

- Have a good repair shop on speed dial. Check with your insurance agent for recommendations. Dealerships are a good choice. An accident or breakdown is not the time to search for a reputable quality garage.

DUI

One in three of us will be involved in a DUI accident in our lifetime. Impaired drivers cause almost half of MVA fatalities, one every 30 minutes. DUI is even higher in accidents and fatalities in age group 16-21. DUI has a staggering cost: $114 billion, of which victims pay $72 billion.

• DUI under 21 – Illegal blood alcohol level is lower. Penalties are far harsher for underage drivers: longer mandatory jail time and 2 year suspension of license.

• DUI over 21 – Expect to go to jail. Depending on your blood alcohol content, you can face felony charges and fines, jail time, mandatory substance abuse treatment, mandatory installation at your expense of vehicle Interlock, community service, lost job and income, and the stigma and lost future income resulting from a permanent criminal record. Court costs alone of $13K are not unusual. Your insurance rates will skyrocket and stay high for years. In addition to the criminal charges, you are exposed to civil liability (rarely covered by your auto insurance) and bankruptcy.

• Don't drink and drive. Use the designated driver plan. Call a sober friend or family member to drive you home. Call a cab. Most clubs will have a standing policy to help patrons who are impaired. Ask the manager.

TRAVEL SAFETY

"One's destination is never a place, but a new way of seeing things."

Henry Miller 1891-1980

Travel Philosophy

Travel expands your cultural, spiritual and intellectual horizons. It exposes you to history and different philosophies, cultures and ways to approach life.

• When in Rome, do as the Romans. While traveling be respectful of people and customs. When traveling abroad, remember it's their country, their culture, their laws.

• Immerse yourself in the culture; be a traveler not a tourist. Do not expect your destination to be like home.

• Good planning makes for a successful trip. Read. Research. Preparation is part of the adventure. Use travel websites like www.tripadvisor.com, www.AAA.com and www.frommers.com.

• Join the AAA. The travel benefits are endless (discounts, maps, insurance, roadside service) and you will have a reputable resource away from home.

• If you have a problem with your travel arrangements, politely ask those responsible for alternatives or if they can find an answer to your problem. You will get a much better response with politeness than rudeness.

• Be vigilant. Crime occurs in vacation destinations just like it does at home.

• Use common sense. Don't do things you wouldn't do at home.

• If it doesn't feel right, don't do it. Follow your instincts.

• Be kind, respectful and courteous with anyone you deal with at your destination and while getting there. You are an ambassador from your town, state and country. Represent them well.

Road Trip

- Plan your trip with Google Maps or AAA. Look at your point to point driving plan, rest and food stops and hotel/motel accommodations.

- Take main highways to get there in a safe and efficient manner. Use the back roads when you want to sightsee, and in daylight only.

- Budget costs of trip (fuel, food, entertainment).

- Get vehicle tuned up by a certified auto mechanic. Check engine, brakes, tires, fluids and electronics.

- Make sure you know how to change a flat tire and/or use the Fix-A-Flat® tire repair product.

- Prepare your vehicle for the trip with water, first aid kit, auto emergency kit, Fix-A-Flat®, healthy snacks, cell phone charger, GPS and paper maps for backup. See Car Emergency Kit.

- Travel during daylight hours. Visibility is the best and emergency services are quicker to respond.

- Take breaks and rotate drivers. If you are tired, stop. Never sleep in your car. Find a hotel or restaurant to rest.

- Never pick up a hitchhiker. No exceptions. You are not in control with a stranger in your car.

- Never stop for someone flagging you down. Instead, call 911 and notify the police of the stranded motorist. If you are physically blocked or stopped, tell them you are calling 911. Call 911 immediately.

- If your car breaks down, stay in your car and lock the doors. Call 911 and/or AAA. If people stop to help, stay in your car and ask them to call AAA or 911 if you do not have a cell phone. Or if you have already called 911, thank them and let them know that AAA and the highway patrol is on the way.

Spring Break

Spring break occurs anytime between February and late April, the most popular destinations are Mexico, Florida, Texas and the Caribbean.

- Many college students today are taking alternative spring break trips to overseas destinations or do community service for charity organizations such as Habitat for Humanity. Not only do these experiences enrich them, but it enhances their resumes for future employment or graduate school. Others use the spring break period to look for summer jobs or internships.

- If you travel for spring break, be aware. At your spring break destination, laws may be stricter and with stiffer penalties than at home. Laws south of the border are severe with regard to public drunkenness, motor vehicle infractions or lewd behavior. Prisons are hellholes, and bail is non-existent.

- Underage drinking, illegal drug use and violence are not legal <u>anywhere</u>.

- Never travel alone on spring break; use a three buddy system if possible. Then if one is in trouble, one can stay with that person and the other can get help. Although Natalee Holloway was with her friends, they did not use the buddy system and she was isolated by her killer. Stay with your buddy.

- Never share details of your hotel, trip itinerary or personal info with new acquaintances. Make a "story" up with your friends that disguises this personal info or just be vague. Practice your "story" so that it is quick and convincing.

- Never leave your drink unattended; always order bottled water or soft drinks. Always get your drink from a bartender. Never accept a drink from a stranger. Criminals will drug victims for robbery, assault and rape.

- If you suspect you have been drugged, immediately call 911 or the local police, request ambulance and police or go directly to the hospital. Ask for a drug screen and stay there until you recover.

- Predators target drunks and the unaware. Don't be a victim.

- Avoid binge drinking. One study found that the average male drinks 18 drinks and the average female drinks 10 drinks per day during spring break. The same study found that 50% of men and 40% of women drank until they were sick or passed out. Vomiting, illness and loss of consciousness are the result of binge drinking.

- Inhibition is a protective mechanism. Loss of inhibition may result in high risk behavior, poor judgment and injury, violence, arrest or worse. Casual, unprotected sex results in STDs and pregnancy. Don't change your moral and ethical standards when you change your latitude.

Travel Health

Foreign travel involves new and different health risks, especially infectious diseases. If you are traveling abroad, see a travel medicine specialist six months before you leave. They are surprisingly efficient and inexpensive. Go to the International Society of Travel Medicine (www.istm.org) to find a doctor who has received the ISTM Certificate in Travel Health™. Get the recommended pre-travel inoculations. Stay up to date; disease prevalence and epidemics are in a constant state of flux.

- Take a first aid kit along with double supply of each prescription medication (store in separate areas).

- Obtain travel health insurance that includes evacuation coverage. This is ridiculously inexpensive and invaluable. No country on earth has health care like the USA.

- Protect your stomach by eating in well established restaurants. Never eat food/drink from street vendors.

- Always wash your hands before eating.

- If you are in the outdoors, use DEET to ward off insects carrying West Nile, Lyme disease, malaria, etc. A concentration of 20-30% is recommended by the CDC. 20% DEET gives you 4 hours of protection while 10% DEET gives you 2 hours of protection. It is not necessary to use a DEET concentration above 30%.

- Be especially careful about driving. Car accidents in foreign countries may cause you to enter a third world healthcare system and if the lack of advanced medicine doesn't kill you, a blood transfusion may (HIV, hepatitis). Use a licensed local driver if overseas, and always insist on a vehicle with seat belts and air bags.

- Do not drink heavily, impairing your judgment.

- Avoid contact that may result in sexually transmitted disease.

- Protect yourself from excessive sun exposure.

- When traveling to the mountains with altitude above 7000 feet, be aware of altitude sickness. Mild: Acute mountain sickness causes headaches, nausea, dizziness and fatigue. Severe: High altitude cerebral and pulmonary edema can be fatal. The higher you travel the more risk.

Check with the CDC websites for health and security alerts prior to traveling overseas.

www.cdc.gov/travel

First Aid Travel Kit

These are items that you should have available to avoid a late night trip to the drugstore or doctor. These travel items should be carried in your car or checked in your luggage (a smaller kit with essentials should be in your carry-on) when traveling.

First Aid Kit and book. Many kits available at drugstores have the basic items including a first aid book. These kits should be augmented with the items below:

- Dual supply of any prescription medicine you normally take (one in the carry-on and the other in checked baggage, so if one is lost the other is available)
- Antibacterial hand sanitizer
- Analgesics (acetaminophen, aspirin or ibuprofen)
- Antacids (Maalox, Zantac or Pepsid)
- Antibiotics (Zpack, Keflex or Cipro)*
- Anti-diarrheal (Pepto-Bismol, Lomitil, Imodium)
- Anti-fungal (Monistat)
- Anti-histamine (Benadryl)
- Topical anti-histamine cream (Benadryl/diphenhydramine)
- Epi-pen (if you have severe allergy to bees, peanuts or other allergens)*
- Laxative
- Sunscreen
- Antibiotic ointment (Bacitracin)
- Hydrocortisone cream
- Eye care items (normal saline drops)
- Band-Aids and tape
- LED flashlight
- Eyeglasses
- Moleskin (for blisters)
- Duct tape
- Scissors, knife and sterile needles
- Antibacterial soap

- Gauze (various sizes)
- Tweezers and safety pin
- J&J Band-Aid Antiseptic Wash
- Ace bandage
- Disposable thermometer
- Bic lighter

* Talk with your physician prior to leaving for recommendations.

Making Airline Reservations

Time spent planning ahead will reap huge rewards in time saved while traveling. Shop online to find the flights with the least number of stops and avoid big hubs in bad weather (mainly winter conditions).

Pearls

- Leave early AM because there are less delays or cancelled flights in the beginning of the travel day. You are more likely to make your connection and get there on time.

- With connecting flights, make the connection time between your flights no less than one hour, and up to two hours. Look at on-time arrival record of your flights when booking.

- Watch the prices in advance. Ticket prices fluctuate depending on how full the plane is and how far out the flight is scheduled.

- Compare ticket price using travel sites such as Orbitz, Expedia or Travelocity; make sure you are getting the best price. www.Kayak.com compares fares and emails you a daily lowest fare.

- Try to make reservations online through the airline's site. You will have more leverage if there is a problem as most other sites are just travel agencies taking a commission.

- If you fly often, consider an airline frequent flyer program to accumulate points and status. Airlines will give you better seats, bump you last and on occasion upgrade you to first class. Obtain credit card from frequent flyer program; you can use points for upgrades or free tickets.

- When calling an airline for reservations, if you're getting nowhere with the representative, politely thank them for their time, hang up and call again. All airline representatives are not created equal.

- Terms: "Direct" means you stay on the same plane with one or more stops, while "Non-Stop" means same plane with no stops.

- Get an aisle seat – easy in/out for bathroom or emergency, more leg room and shoulder room.

- Sit near the midsection exit row, the front exit row or the bulkhead. Whether in an emergency or just getting off the plane in a timely fashion, it is best to be near an exit. Bulkhead and exit rows have more legroom. Seats in front of the exit row and in the exit row usually do not recline. If it's a long flight sit behind the exit row or two in front.

- Avoid seats in the very rear of the plane. If equipment is changed, rows 1 through 24 are usually on all jet aircraft, but not rows 25-67. And the air is better up front; less carbon dioxide and away from the toilet.

- Go to www.seatguru.com for a look at the best seat on your particular flight and plane.

- Take your government issued ID card and the credit card you bought the ticket with to the airport; you can use it to check in at the kiosk.

- <u>Never buy a ticket without a seat assignment</u>. Always be sure that you get assigned a seat when you buy a ticket. If a seat assignment is unavailable, it may be an overbooked flight. You are the last one in line and may not get a seat. If this is the only flight for you, then call the airline every day until you get an assigned seat (people cancel their tickets).

- Check in online at home within 24 hours of flight. You can get your boarding pass and confirm your seats, upgrade, pay for your luggage at a reduced rate and have everything ready (except baggage check-in) prior to leaving for the airport, all in the comfort of your home.

- Save a copy of your e-ticket in your email, laptop or smartphone so you can access your itinerary or ticket as needed.

Before You Leave

Create an itinerary that documents your trip with dates, schedule, flights, travel route, hotel and contact phone numbers. Print this and give it to one or two trusted adults who will know to keep it confidential. Email, blogs, and other social media posting of travel plans have resulted in burglary and worse. No one should know of your travel until you return.

Preparing to Leave

- Obtain travel cash and a prepaid debit card. If you plan to use your ATM, check your bank balance before leaving and inform the bank of your travel plans.

- Carry your cash and credit cards in different spots. Put a hidden stash of cash and a copy of your driver's license or passport in your luggage or carry-on, in case you are robbed.

- If you are going overseas, contact your cell phone carrier and upgrade to an international plan.

- Bring first aid kit, medications and antibacterial wipes. Pack your own pillow or pillow encasement.

- Pack smart and travel light, choose multi-use clothing. Pack your shoes in plastic bags to keep clothes clean.

- Place your important medicines and valuables in your carry-on luggage. Do not bring expensive jewelry, electronics or anything that you can't afford to lose. Furthermore, flashy items attract attention and criminals.

- Buy timers and set lights and/or a radio to go on during the evening. Make sure they are not near any flammable items (curtains, papers). Leave an outside light on.

- Ask a trusted neighbor to watch your home, pick up unexpected packages, etc. Cancel your newspaper and hold your mail.

- Check that the stove, oven and water are turned off. Shut the main water valve off to prevent a small leak from becoming a disaster.

- Unplug computer, electronics, low voltage transformers and television. Unplug coffee maker and other appliances. These are all fire hazards.

- Empty the garbage.

- Lock all windows and doors, shut blinds in bedrooms and turn designated lights on.

- Before leaving do a final walk through.

Airline Travel Basics

Airline travel in the aftermath of 9/11 is complicated and stressful. Good preparation beforehand and consideration for other travelers during the journey will go a long way in making the experience more enjoyable.

- Review your tickets 48 hours in advance and call or check online to confirm times. Do this again the morning before you leave for the airport.

- Check in online, usually 24 hours prior to your flight. Print two boarding passes; put one in your carry-on and the other in your wallet.

- Remember to dress with limited metal objects (belt buckle, jewelry, body piercing or metal buttons), as these will activate the metal detector at the TSA security check point. Wear comfortable clothes and easily removed shoes; you will be taking your shoes off in security.

- When going through security, be patient but alert. Take your shoes off and take items out of pockets in advance. Put your valuables through last, right before you go through the metal detector. Keep them in your sight at all times.

- TSA uses two types of full body scan devices: the grey millimeter wave scanner (ProVision) and the blue Castscope X-ray scanner (Rapiscan). Avoid the Castscope X-ray machine, if possible. This machine uses low radiation (10 µRem) to screen passengers. Although the level is low, it is best to avoid the exposure. Typical x-ray machines emit 10,000 to 100,000 µRem.

- Keep any medications, food, candy, etc. in clear zip seal bags. This allows TSA personnel to view without touching. The blue gloves TSA uses are for their protection, not yours; the gloves get filthy touching travelers, baggage and shoes.

- Place identification on outside and inside of baggage. Use your first initial and last name (conceal your gender), city, state, USA and cell phone number. Use your or your parent's office address if possible. Do not put your home address on your luggage or travel documents.

- Never travel with expensive luggage. This merely entices and invites criminals: Expensive luggage implies expensive contents.

- Always use TSA approved locks. Any others may be cut off.

- To identify your bags, place unique stickers, colored duct tape or painted markings on outside of the bag. Most bags look the same on the baggage carousel.

- Check your baggage requirements (size and weight) before leaving home. Check your airline's carry-on rules. Weigh your bag. Expect your bag to be searched.

- Arrive at least 2 hours before domestic flight and 3 hours before international flight. Be at the gate 45 minutes prior to departure.

- Be prepared with ticket and ID (passport if international) at the airline check-in counter and security.

- Do not stand near the x-ray machine for extended periods of time (limit potential radiation exposure).

- Confirm on the Departures/Arrivals board when your flight leaves and from what gate. On time? Boarding time? Gate change?

- Go to the gate and verify flight. If changed, ask the gate agent where your flight is departing from.

- It is a good idea to purchase bottled water once through security. Ice and water from the airplane galley have been shown to be contaminated with bacteria. Hydration is important, and water is the best choice.

- Wait in the boarding area until called and then board in order. However, try to be first in your group as the overhead compartments fill up fast.

Infectious Disease on Planes

Mass transit, whether it is airplane, bus, train or ship, places you in direct contact with many people and many new contagious diseases. Often you will be stressed, tired and dehydrated. These factors increase your exposure and susceptibility to disease at the worst possible place and time. Bear in mind that disease causing viruses can survive for days on smooth surfaces. Fortunately, there are several little things you can do to greatly diminish your risk.

- Check-in Kiosks – Have been touched by thousands of dirty hands. Use them carefully and then use hand sanitizer immediately afterward.

- TSA Bins – Remember that people's shoes have been in them, which have tracked through bathrooms and on sidewalks.

- Water – Airplane water sources have been found to have fecal bacteria, as has ice. Once through TSA, purchase bottled water for the trip.

- Beverages – Attempt to purchase a full can of beverage, and drink without ice.

- Tray Tables – People do disgusting things on tray tables, including changing diapers. Studies show a high contamination rate for the potentially fatal MRSA in all three major airlines; never touch with open wound. Consider bringing an antiseptic wipe to clean the table. Be careful not to touch the tray and then your face or beverage or snack.

- Never travel with an open wound. Use liquid bandage and Band-Aids on all hand/arm/face cuts, however minor, before travel.

- Seatback Pouch – Fecal bacteria, used tissues, gum, other contaminated waste. Avoid.

- Pillows & Blankets – Who used them last, and for what? They can harbor bacteria, viruses and mold.

- Airplane Toilets – Contaminated. The high pressure vacuum flush system sprays aerosol droplets of fecal matter and waste in the air, effectively coating the interior of the lavatory. Seat, handles, sink and switches are colonized. This has been linked to spread of H1N1, SARS and MRSA. Use the lavatory quickly and wash hands using proper technique. See Hand Washing. Use a paper towel to turn faucet handles and open door. Then use hand sanitizer when your return to your seat. Never brush your teeth in the lavatory.

On the Plane

You are all on the plane together, you are all getting there at the same time, and you will all be deplaning and meeting again at baggage and in the parking lot. Be civil and considerate. Rudeness will be rewarded in kind.

• Be patient when boarding. Follow airline protocol.

• After boarding, find your seat and promptly store your bags at your feet or overhead. Don't block the aisle.

• Look for the emergency exits, count the number of rows (in a smoke filled cabin, you may not be able to see the exit signs). Plan your exit.

• Every hour, drink bottled water or juice without ice (bacteria are often present in ice and onboard water sources). Avoid alcohol, caffeine, soft drinks or coffee; all are diuretics which dehydrate you.

• Eat light when offered airline food. Bring your own healthy snacks and drink bottled water purchased after clearing TSA security.

• Bring a book, music or magazines to entertain yourself.

• Do in seat exercises (wiggle your toes, move your feet and stretch your legs). These maneuvers are often described in airline magazines. Get up and walk the cabin every two hours to increase circulation, minimize swelling and possible blood clot formation in your legs.

• Talk with your doctor about other precautions such as wearing elastic compression stockings for long flights and/or taking a baby aspirin before flight if you are at risk for blood clots (smokers, birth control pills, recent surgery or injury, obesity).

• Go to the restroom before leaving the airport. If you have to use the airplane bathroom, avoid excessive hand contact with knobs and faucets. Turn around, lower lid and face door when flushing toilet to avoid aerosol spray in face. Use hand sanitizer upon returning to your seat.

• Do not get up during drink/food service. This is a safety issue and an inconvenience to the flight attendants and everyone around you.

• Dress appropriately. Wear long pants and shirts (airline seats are not cleaned often). Wear cotton; it does not burn or melt like polyester or synthetics. Wear flat shoes with non-gripping soles that you can run in for emergencies and they will not catch on the inflatable emergency exit ramp. Do not wear open toed shoes or sandals.

- If asked by a passenger to switch seats, simply state "I'm sorry, but I'd like to stay here." If you wish to switch, only switch after doors are closed, head count is complete and crew permits moving.

- When reclining your seat, move it slowly.

- Stay within your space, share armrests, watch your feet.

- Do not grab the back of the seat in front of you when getting up or use seat backs like a jungle gym to climb or walk through the aisle.

- If you are late for a connecting plane, tell the flight attendants. They may be able to help you disembark or notify the gate.

- Disembark in an orderly fashion, row by row, in order. Be polite.

- Go immediately to baggage and identify your bag as it comes off the conveyer belt. Have your luggage claim stubs handy.

Terminals are secure and safe. It's a good policy to regroup, organize and plan before leaving the terminal, especially in foreign lands. Gather your possessions and, if unsure, check with the information booth/airport authorities/security as to where you need to go (rental cars, official taxi stand or passenger pickup). Then proceed outside the terminal.

Taxicabs

Taxicabs are a quick and easy means of transportation in the big city, at home or abroad. They are also the best transportation if you have consumed alcohol or are impaired. Sometimes the trip can be a cross between an amusement park ride and a demolition derby, so take care in selecting your cab and always buckle up.

- Always use reputable cab companies. Ask at your hotel concierge, front desk, bar or restaurant staff.

- When arriving at an airport, always go to a taxi stand and obtain a registered taxi. Unlicensed drivers will often pretend to be cab drivers to pick up tourists and overcharge or rob their passengers.

- American cabs are metered and regulated. Make sure the meter is on zero when you enter the cab and that the cab driver starts the meter at the beginning your ride.

- Avoid fixed prices unless you have discussed the price with the hotel doorman or front desk, and that this is fair and legal in this locale (i.e. some cities have a fixed rate from airport to city center).

- You can negotiate your fare, but this must be done prior to getting in the cab. Talk to the cabbie from the sidewalk.

- When you call for a cab, avoid others overhearing your plans. Get the name of the driver and color of cab that will be picking you up.

- When dining in a local restaurant, ask the host or hostess to call a cab. Pay your bill and wait at the table until your cab has arrived.

- Try to share a cab with a friend. Avoid solo rides.

- Always sit in the back seat.

- Never approach a cab; have the cab come to you. Visually inspect the cab and driver before getting in. Talk with the driver before getting in. Tell him where you want to go and ask what the fare will be. Do not be shy about rejecting a cab. Simply pretend you got a cell phone call and say that you have changed your plans. Better safe than sorry.

- When you get in take a photo with your phone, write down his name and license (let the driver know you are doing this) or ask for a card from the driver. If you have a complaint, compliment or forget something in the cab, you have his name and cab number. Of course, this will also deter criminal activity if he knows he has been photographed.

- Ask the driver to take you on the shortest, cheapest route. You can use your smartphone GPS to confirm that he is taking you by the most direct route.

- Tipping cab drivers is usually 15% in the US and abroad.

- Pay and receive change before exiting the cab.

- If your driver and you have a fare dispute, put the amount of money you feel is fair on the seat next to you and get out. Contact the authorities if you feel you have been threatened.

Public Transportation

Urban mass transit is buses, subways and trains. They are efficient, convenient, economical and green. When using mass transit, investigate the options and reputation in your area. You will be riding with all of society, both good and bad. Vigilance is important.

- Obtain a multiple day pass if available.

- Travel during peak hours when there are many passengers. Avoid the evening hours.

- Travel with a buddy. Blend into the crowd. Do not make it obvious you are tourists or novice riders.

- Be alert for pick-pockets and purse-snatchers. Put your wallet in your front pocket and your purse across your shoulder and chest, not hanging off your shoulder. Hold on to it.

- Get off in areas where there are many people, not at a desolate stop.

- Sit in a window seat with items of value against the wall.

- Never wear expensive clothing or jewelry on mass transit. Dress for the situation. If you have a party or event that requires fine attire, take a cab.

- Be wary of strangers. If someone is giving you unsolicited advice, is overly friendly or inquisitive, be alert. Answer questions in a polite, disinterested way and move on. (See Patterned Response).

Hotel Reservations and Check-in

To seasoned travelers, their hotel is their sanctuary. They select hotels with good locations, top amenities and excellent service. There is merit in choosing the best accommodations your budget will allow; online booking allows you to see your hotel, read reviews and get competitive rates. A little research will get you the hotel that meets all your expectations, with no unpleasant surprises. www.tripadvisor.com is a travel website with candid reviews and photos from other travelers. You can also use www.frommers.com and www.fodors.com to study your destination for the best accommodations, events, restaurants and sites.

- Pick a hotel in a busy, safe area of town. The newer the hotel, the better the security system will be. Choose a hotel with a small contained lobby or one main entrance so that the hotel security can deter loitering.

- Hotels with interior atriums are excellent choices as all the rooms are visible from the hallways (example: Embassy Suites).

- Reserve your room as "Mr. and Mrs. J. Smith" or "J. Smith". Use your first initial and last name, never your first name, so as not to identify your gender. There is usually no extra charge for two in a room and it gives the illusion that you are not alone.

- Use hotels with electronic door locks. The combination on the magnetic card is changed with each guest and if you lose your key, the card can be reprogrammed.

- Try to find hotels with room safes or safety deposit boxes at reception. Valuables are not safe in your hotel room.

- Request a room that is on the 2nd floor to 6th floor; 7th floor and above may not be within reach of the typical 100 foot fire ladder. Ground floor rooms are more easily entered by criminals.

- If you are alone, request a room that is near the elevator and not at the end of the hallway, near stairwells or a long walk from elevator. These rooms are more public and safer.

- When checking in, never announce your room number or allow the clerk to announce your number. Ask for two keys, one for you and one for your fictitious "spouse/guest/brother".

- If alone, consider using a bellman to escort you to your room. Wait outside the door until the bellman has turned on the lights and placed your luggage. Have the money ready and do not open your wallet or purse in front of the bellman. Give the tip at the door.

- Avoid stairwell; take the elevator. When entering an elevator with others, be the last one to enter your floor number. If someone in the elevator makes you uncomfortable, get off in public area (lobby) or with other passengers.

In Your Hotel Room

Great accommodations can be a relaxing, rejuvenating experience after a journey. Settle in, explore and enjoy your new environment, but remember to maintain your personal vigilance and stay safe.

- Security at major hotel chains is good, but there are still risks. Travelers are vulnerable, and criminals exploit this. You are in their territory and unlikely to return to press charges or appear at trial. Prevention is the best strategy.

- Always deadbolt your room. Get in the habit of doing this <u>immediately</u> upon entering. Carry a rubber door stopper or door stop alarm to place under the door when locked, preventing unwanted intruders. There are many master keys in hotels.

- Use an antibacterial wipe to clean the remote control, telephone, drinking glasses (followed by hot water), light switches, plumbing fixtures and door handles to rid your room of unwanted bacteria and viruses.

- Inspect the bed, sheets and general cleanliness of the room. Check for bedbugs and their brown streaks. Change rooms if you are not happy.

- Sleep in long sleeved shirts and long pants for barrier protection.

- Use your own pillow or bring a pillow barrier encasement to block dust mites, mold and allergens. Pillows do not get washed. Secretions from the last guest may still be on that pillow.

- Check that the balconies are not so close that someone can jump from one to the next; if so, ask for another room or secure the window or sliding glass door.

- Keep curtains closed, TV on and lights on when you are in the room and while you are out.

- Read <u>Fire Exit</u> information on the door. Note the number of doors you are away from exit (in a fire you will not be able to see well). Note location of fire alarm and extinguisher.

- If there is a fire, check that the door is not hot before opening. Stay low with wet towel over face. If you cannot leave room, fill bath tub with cold water, block bottom of door with wet towels, unlock door and chain, stay low to the floor. If it's too hot and you are unable to leave then enter the tub.

- Carry a LED flashlight in case of fire or power outage.

- Do not throw anything in trash that identifies you (baggage tags, receipts, etc.). Take with you and shred.

- Never accept unexpected deliveries or open door for hotel personnel (unless you have confirmed with front desk the reason for the personnel's presence at your room).

- When ordering room service: Meet waiter at door with pen in hand, stay at open door and instruct the waiter to place food just inside room, sign at the open door and then close and lock.

- Meet visitors in the lobby and not your room. Do not tell strangers your room number.

- Never say your room number at front desk, restaurants or in lobby. Write or show key to identify your room number. This is for personal security and to avoid fraudulent charges to your room. If you are alone, pay with credit card in restaurant/shops rather than with a room charge.

- Do not leave valuables, laptop or smartphone in your room unsecured. Take them with you or use the hotel safety deposit box or the room safe.

When you leave, gather all your belongings then double check the room, closet, shower and drawers. Don't forget your pillow or pillow encasement. Keep a key in the event you leave something behind.

Preparing for Overseas Travel

Travel anywhere but within the US now requires a passport. Even if you have no immediate travel plans, acquire a US passport. Forms are at the US Post Office, take a month or more to process, and are good for ten years.

- Be aware that some countries require a visa for entry. Without one you may be detained at the port of entry. Visas take time to obtain. Plan in advance.

- Go to the US State Department site www.travel.state.gov for country specific information such as visa requirements, warnings, registration with US Embassy, etc.

- Go to the Centers for Disease Control www.cdc.gov/travel for information on recommended or required immunizations and medications.

- For health warnings go to www.cdc.gov/travel or www.who.int.

- Call your health insurance provider and find out if you are covered in the countries you visit. If not, obtain medical travel and evacuation insurance. This can be obtained from your insurance broker, American Express or your travel agent.

- If you plan to drive, learn the rules of the road for your destination. Be especially careful in countries that drive on the left side of the road. Years of driving on the right can lead to tragedy. Never drink and drive.

- Obtain a money belt or secret pouch for important documents and cash.

- Check with your cell phone company and add on international phone, text and data service.

- Use a temporary email address (yahoo, gmail or site of choice) for contact with friends and family. Internet cafes are not secure and you can dump the email address when you get home.

- Get two prescriptions of every medicine you take (carry one and pack the other). Make an updated medication list and medical history for your trip.

- Make copies of your passport, driver's license, credit cards, medical history and itinerary. Leave one at home and carry the other in a secret pocket. If you can, scan your passport and email a copy to yourself and family/friend at home.

- Travel light and pack sensibly. Use items of clothing that do not wrinkle, are multipurpose, and can be washed/dried quickly. Synthetic/poly blends work best. www.rei.com.

Obtain a Frommer's, Fodor's or Lonely Planet travel book for your destination. Read about your country and take the book with you. If it is a large book, cut out the sections that you need and leave the rest at home. Buy a phrase book/CD to learn the local language, even a few phrases will endear you to the locals. Blend into the local life and try not to be the stereotypical tourist, but rather a traveler and adventurer. You will be safer and gain greater access to the culture and experience.

Safety in Public and Traveling

Crime occurs everywhere, and whether you are traveling in the US or foreign countries, you are a potential target for criminals. They know that you are unfamiliar with your surroundings, vulnerable and usually in a carefree frame of mind with your guard down. Furthermore, they know it is unlikely that you will file charges or return as a witness in a trial.

• <u>Maintain a 360° situational awareness at all times in public</u>. Frequently look over your shoulder. Make brief, non-threatening eye contact.

• Keep your money, credit cards, documents, passport and debit cards in your wallet, purse or money belt, not in a fanny pack. The money belt is the best option and easy to wear once you get used to it. We recommend a belt loop money belt for ease of access and comfort. www.magellans.com.

• Leave copies of all documents you are carrying with a relative at home.

• When walking on sidewalks, stay in the <u>center</u> of the sidewalk. People rush out of doorways without looking, or with packages in their arms. Criminals may lurk in doorways.

• Keep your purse on the side away from the street to avoid a motorcycle thief grabbing your purse from the road. This is a common tactic abroad.

• When in restaurants, keep your purse at your feet or on your lap, not on the back of the chair.

• When approaching an alley, pause and look. Cars backing out have poor visibility, and muggers may lurk there.

• Sightseeing: This is particularly vulnerable time. Your attention is distracted, and this is the time assailants prefer to act.

• Always maintain a safety zone around yourself. Things happen fast.

Street People

Do not talk to soliciting strangers. You may be approached by panhandlers, beggars, scam artists and hustlers. They all want your money. Immediately tell them "No Thank You!" loudly and firmly, and back away, reaching for your cell phone. Engaging them in polite chat only encourages them, establishes rapport and allows them to get closer to you physically.

See Patterned Response. If they persist, call 911 or authorities.

Outdoor Adventures

Few experiences equal the majesty and splendor of the great outdoors. If you are a novice, begin in our National Parks or one of the many state parks and advance to the more remote areas after gaining knowledge of the outdoors. Proper, quality gear and preparation is critical. Great adventures turning sour are usually due to poor planning, overconfidence or underestimating nature.

Preparation

- Research the area beforehand. Go online, read, call the site and talk with the Park Ranger or camp site representative. Look at satellite and topo maps. Use Google Maps and Google Earth.

- Know the weather, terrain, animal population and park services at your planned destination.

- Know your limits; are you a novice or an Eagle Scout? Tailor your trip to your experience. Ask outfitters or Park Rangers for recommendations.

- Set the length of time based on your experience in the outdoors. If you are a novice, then start with one or two nights camping.

- Have the proper gear for the area. Check with a local outfitter for recommendations. Is drinkable water available? What is the terrain like? How far is the hike? Temperature fluctuations? Do I need foul weather gear?

- Have a detailed checklist of supplies, food, water, water purification, maps, permits, reservations and safety gear. Go to www.rei.com/expertadvice for more info.

- Stay hydrated and drink only purified water. Purified water is water that has been treated for viruses, bacteria and cysts. Filtered water has been treated for bacteria and cysts; viruses will travel through the filter. Filtered water must be further treated with iodine or chlorine bleach to kill viruses.

- Review maps of the area before camping or hiking. Carry a compass or GPS, whistle and signal mirror with you at all times. Learn how to navigate with a map and compass in the woods.

- Check weather before leaving home.

- Bring a travel first aid kit.

- Send your itinerary to friends or family. Check in with the Park Ranger and give itinerary when backpacking.

- If you are not near a Park Service office then leave an itinerary of your trip in your car. Search and rescue personnel will look in your car first and your itinerary will help in the effort to find you.

Lost in the Outdoors

S.T.O.P. **S**tay Calm, **T**hink, **O**bserve, **P**lan.

<u>Stay Calm</u>. Stop and sit down. Drink and Eat. Check what you have with you.

<u>Think</u>. Evaluate where you are, look at map, recall your path, look at the topography.

<u>Observe</u>. Look for paths, footprints, buildings, smoke, highways, clearings, weather or local shelter. Listen for sounds of civilization.

<u>Plan</u>. If you know where you are, plot a course home. Use a compass if you have one. Mark your path with rocks or branches so that you know if you are going in a circle and so that rescuers notice your trail.

The Basics

- Stay put. If you do not know where you are, don't waste energy wandering. They will find you. You can survive several days without water and weeks without food.

- Hunker down. Find shelter under a tree or large rock, start a fire, stay warm and dry, ration your food and water.

- Make your distress signal in the highest, clearest spot possible.

- Add green leaves or grass to the fire to make smoke to attract aircraft, or use a mirror or glass to reflect the sun. Work your whistle.

- Hang bright colored clothing to attract rescue.

- Your cell phone can be used to locate you. Turn the phone off until needed so as to conserve battery power. Find high ground for best signal and call 911 first, <u>not home</u>; your battery life is limited. VHF radios are line of sight, but may help to talk with rescuers. Consider a satellite phone for remote areas. Satellite phone rentals are convenient, affordable, and function from anywhere on the globe.

Universal Distress Signals

Radio or Phone Signals

Low Urgency: <u>PanPan</u> indicates breakdown, stranded.

High Urgency: <u>MayDay</u> indicates life threatening situation.

SOS Morse Code: <u>dot dot dot</u> <u>dash dash dash</u> <u>dot dot dot</u>

Visual and Ground To Air Signals

Three Signal Fires: In a triangle, 50 feet apart.

Triangle of rocks or bright fabrics, 50 feet apart.

Audible Signals

Loud Noise (yell, whistle, gunshot, horn) <u>three times in a row</u>.

Radio Protocols and Distress Signals

There will be times when you will need to use a radio to communicate, whether you are on the water, hiking, outdoors or in emergency situations. Handheld FRS, GMRS, CB radios and VHF marine radios function differently from a phone. <u>Only one person can talk at a time</u>. Additionally, transmission strength and clarity are subject to distance and atmospheric influences. Therefore, protocols exist so that messages are not lost, misunderstood or overtalked.

Channels: Radios use specific frequency bands and within each band there are multiple channels. Certain channels are priority/emergency and monitored by authorities and rescue personnel. These channels are not to be used for routine communication. They are used to make contact and then <u>switch</u> to another channel to talk. Never conduct a conversation on a priority channel. You may be blocking an emergency call. Channel 16 Marine VHF is the priority channel for hailing, weather and distress calls only.

Realize that radio transmissions are open and are monitored by the public as they can be a source of great amusement as well as news, weather, and events.

<u>PTT Push To Talk/Release To Listen</u>: Radios have a small PTT button that will be pressed to begin talking. Once finished with your message, release the button. Keep your thumb off the PTT button all other times. Pushing the PTT button while the other person is talking will block all communication. Talk slowly and clearly to be understood. Speak in a normal voice. Yelling only causes distortion. Do not speak directly into the microphone, but across it. Keep messages short and precise.

Squelch: Attenuates radio static. Turn knob up until static is loud, then back it off until quiet.

Radio Protocol

Sound Check: Transmission quality is rated by strength and clarity on a scale of 5. A strong and clear message is rated: 5 x 5 or <u>Loud and Clear</u>. A poor rating might be 3 x 2.

- Numbers: For clarity, say "one-six", not "sixteen".

- Repeat all critical information for clarity.

- Affirmative: Yes.

- Negative: No.

- Roger: Message received.

- WilCo: <u>Wil</u>l <u>Co</u>mply (with message received).

- Say Again: Repeat last message.

- Standby or Wait One: Pause. You should remain on channel, but be quiet.

- Over: Indicates message completed, and reply expected.

- Out: Indicates message completed and no reply expected.

- Clear: Indicates that you're finished talking and will shut off radio.

Distress Call Protocol

<u>Break-Break</u>: Alert to all listeners that a distress or emergency call is to follow.

<u>Sécurité, Sécurité, Sécurité</u>: Maritime urgent call, non-life threatening.

<u>Pan-Pan, Pan-Pan, Pan-Pan</u>: Maritime/General distress call, usually indicates breakdown or moderate threat to life.

<u>Mayday, Mayday, Mayday</u>: Maritime/General distress call indicating vessel in danger, or life in imminent danger. This call has priority over all calls.

NATO Alphabet

The NATO and US military phonetic alphabet is very useful in phone, radio and other communication where clarity is essential. Each word used is distinctive and easily understood by the listener. Civilian use is widespread as well, and especially valuable for giving email addresses, and in phone conversations.

- A: Alpha
- B: Bravo
- C: Charlie
- D: Delta
- E: Echo
- F: Foxtrot
- G: Golf
- H: Hotel
- I: India
- J: Juliet
- K: Kilo
- L: Lima
- M: Mike
- N: November
- O: Oscar
- P: Papa
- Q: Quebec
- R: Romeo
- S: Sierra
- T: Tango
- U: Uniform
- V: Victor
- W: Whiskey
- X: X-ray
- Y: Yankee
- Z: Zulu

KEYS TO SUCCESS

"Nothing is less important than which fork you use. Etiquette is the science of living. It embraces everything. It is ethics. It is honor."

Emily Post 1872-1960

Etiquette

America is a very young and egalitarian society, unlike other cultures that may have millennia of tradition and arcane customs. While our rules of etiquette have been relaxed in the last century, proper manners are still a hallmark of sophistication. Proper etiquette and good manners is more than a guide to coexisting harmoniously and elegantly; they show consideration of others. Courtesy is not a restriction of freedom of expression, but a way to distinguish oneself in a positive light in business, social and romantic settings, because good manners, like common sense, are uncommon.

Special Note to Male Readers:

American culture glorifies machismo exploits, and etiquette and manners are considered effete or a sign of weakness by some people. It is probably truer that rudeness is a sign of ignorance, not power. Rather, a polite and courteous manner conveys a quiet strength as exemplified by world class professional boxer, Olympic medalist and former undisputed middleweight champion, Jermain Taylor. His serene, respectful interviews after brutal prize fights personify grace and elegance in a warrior who need bow to no man.

"Rudeness is the weak man's imitation of strength"

Eric Hoffer 1902-1983

The Cardinal Rules of Etiquette

If you only follow these seven rules, you will be far ahead of the vast majority of humanity. Etiquette evolves, and some rules such as men removing hats while indoors have questionable modern validity. However, the following rules will never change:

1. Do not overtalk (begin speaking while another is speaking) or interrupt.

2. Do not talk with food in your mouth.

3. Do not chew with your mouth open.

4. Do not groom publicly: Pick nose, ears, teeth, and so on.

5. Be Punctual. There is no such thing as "fashionably late". Lateness is always rude.

6. Never discuss: <u>Sex, Religion or Politics</u>. These topics are strongly held, emotionally charged, and not always subject to logic or rational discourse.

7. RSVP when requested. And honor it. RSVP means *Repondez, S'il Vous Plait;* French for "Reply, if you please." The host or hostess will plan and buy for the expected number of guests. Not responding is not only rude but wastes the host's money and time in preparation. And never show up unexpectedly.

Basic Etiquette

These are the basics rules of ètiquette and good manners. They can make or break a deal, relationship or interview. Master them, doors will open; ignore them, doors will close.

• Always use "Please", "Thank you" and "Excuse me".

• Always smile when greeting another person. It sets the mood.

• When meeting, use a firm hand shake and eye contact.

• Stand and sit up straight.

• Compliment sincerely. Look for the good in everyone.

• Do not interrupt.

• Answer when spoken to.

• Use a normal tone of voice. Never yell or talk loudly.

• Do not curse or use vulgar language.

• Never get angry. Control the situation.

• Eat slowly and chew with your mouth closed.

• Burping and flatulence should never occur in public.

• Dipping snuff or chewing tobacco in public is impolite.

• Dress for the occasion. If in doubt dress up, not down.

• Avoid extreme, controversial or provocative clothing.

• Write "Thank You" notes when receiving gifts, meeting an important person or staying at someone's home. Mail them. Email is not a substitute.

• Open doors for others, entering and exiting.

• Help the elderly, young children and others not as fortunate as you.

• Never groom in public: Adjusting, scratching, picking, applying makeup, combing hair, cleaning or clipping nails, toothpick use, etc. in public is crude. Refrain or go to the restroom.

• Expect to be treated with courtesy. Avoid those who do not treat you with respect.

Greetings

- Proper Greeting: "Good Morning/Afternoon/Evening" or "Hello".

- Show respect to elders, employers/supervisors, teachers, religious leaders or others worthy of a more formal greeting.

- The handshake is the customary western greeting (some cultures do not shake hands as it is considered offensive). The handshake should be firm, not flaccid or crushing. Look the person in the eye and shake (not pump) their hand. Try to equal the firmness of the person's hand you are shaking. Do not give women a limp handshake. This can be considered insulting.

- Limit touching, kissing or hugging casual acquaintances. This sends the wrong signal. Reserve it for family and close friends.

- When kissing relatives or close friends, start on the right cheek first. Make a definite move and heads will not collide.

- When making an introduction, look at both parties as you introduce them. Use formal names with formal introductions (Mr./Mrs./Ms./Dr.) and first names with informal introductions. Introduce both parties to each other (Mr. Jones, I'd like you to meet Dr. Smith; Dr. Smith this is my teacher, Mr. Jones).

- When you are being introduced to someone, listen and repeat the name. "It's nice to meet you, Dr. Smith." Repetition helps you remember their name.

- If you have forgotten someone's name after being introduced, don't panic. This is common. Quickly apologize and ask. "I'm so sorry, could you repeat your name."

- If you have forgotten someone's name when you are introducing them, apologize and say you have gone blank and forgotten their name.

- If someone forgets to introduce you, politely introduce yourself: "Hello, my name is James West."

- When finishing your conversation, say "Goodbye" not "Bye" or "Later". If the conversation is going too long, tell the person, "I wish I did not have to go. It has been great seeing you. We will have to get together soon." Finish on a positive note.

Telephone Etiquette

Phones and cell phones are ubiquitous and part of daily life. The following are basic rules of etiquette for phones.

Calling

- Dial carefully; if you misdial, apologize. Remember that wrong numbers waste a stranger's time and money, and that they will have your number.
- Never call before 8AM or after 9PM. Avoid mealtimes.
- Do not call near the end of business hours or closing time.
- Never call with food, gum, candy, etc. in your mouth.
- When they answer, immediately identify yourself: "Hello, this is ___ ."
- No computer surfing, TV, eating while on a call.

Answering the Phone

- "Hello" is the proper response. Let them identify themselves.
- For unwanted sales calls, say politely "No, thank you." If they call again, ask to be placed on the National Do Not Call Registry, www.donotcall.gov. See Patterned Response.

General Rules

- Call Waiting: Ask before putting someone on hold. Speak briefly with the new caller and get back to your original call within ten seconds.
- Don't be rude on the phone. You are not anonymous any more.
- Don't slam or drop the receiver. This can hurt the caller's ear.
- Keep conversations brief and concise with busy people.
- If using a speakerphone, tell the other party immediately.
- When using a cell phone, keep a ten foot radius as you talk and do not have loud, emotional public conversations.
- Return calls and voicemail in a prompt fashion.
- Phone use during class, work or situations such as concerts, movies or conferences is unacceptable. Personal calls in classroom settings are disruptive, in group situations inconsiderate, and while at work can be a cause for termination. Take the call at a later, appropriate time.

Special Situations

When dealing with customer service reps about a consumer/business issue, always get their first and last name or ID number immediately. If service is poor, ask to speak with their supervisor. Endeavor to speak only with someone who has the power to resolve your problem. Make notes including date and time. Move up the chain of command until the issue is resolved.

Tape Recording Telephone Conversations – In many states it is legal to record your own conversations without notifying the other party. This is easy to do, and can be invaluable in legal or business disputes. Check your laws before recording.

Internet Etiquette

- Realize that you are <u>not</u> anonymous or untraceable. Your IP address is digitally imprinted on every internet move you make, every site you visit, every email or IM or post you make. You can be found.

- Consider all internet communications to be public. Once it's out there, it's out there forever.

- Do not post anything on social media you wouldn't want your entire family seeing.

- Do not let the impersonal nature of the internet affect your etiquette; you are still communicating with real people.

- Do not write on the internet what you would not say in person.

- Remember all correspondence, including emails, IM/Chat conversations and forum comments can be copied, stored, forwarded and printed.

- Use proper salutations in your email.

- Respond to emails in a prompt and timely fashion.

- Use proper grammar and sentence form.

- Avoid abbreviations (u, r, 2, etc.) in communications.

- Do not use all CAPS. This connotes anger or yelling.

- Never use vulgarity.

- Never flame (a rude email or IM reply) or respond to other posts or profiles.

- Never post provocative or sexually explicit photographs of yourself or others. It is a public domain and others will view those pictures.

- Do not send chain letters or cc: every joke you find. This is a common tactic to transmit hidden viruses or worms.

- Never open or respond to junk mail.

- Never click on <u>hyperlinks</u> in emails, especially unknown senders.

Dining Etiquette

Proper table manners are a cornerstone of civilized society. They are easy to learn, simple to practice, and establish a level of polish and sophistication few other trappings of culture can exceed.

- Pull the chair out for your female guests. Sit after the ladies are seated.

- When you sit down, take the napkin and place it in your lap. It stays in your lap during the meal. Convention is to place napkin on chair if you leave the table; however, this is unsanitary. We recommend it is placed on the table. When the meal is done, it is placed on the table to the left of your plate, never on the plate.

- Do not use the napkin as a handkerchief or toothbrush.

- Do not text or talk on the phone during a meal. Leave the table if you have an urgent phone call.

- Do not scratch your head or rub any part of your body during your meal.

- Know which utensils and plates are yours (see Table Settings).

- Begin to eat after your host or date begins the meal.

- Chew with your mouth closed.

- Do not speak with food in your mouth.

- Sit up straight and look your dining companions in the eye.

- No elbows on the table, only your hands or forearms are allowed.

- Use polite conversation with no interrupting, argumentative subjects or foul language. Avoid inflammatory topics: Sex, Religion, Politics.

- Do not inhale your meal. Enjoy the meal. Americans eat in a rush; Europeans eat slowly and savor the food and the experience. There is evidence that this may explain the lower incidence of obesity in Europe.

Table Settings

Few of us routinely encounter a full place setting, continental style. However, when one does, it is a sign of polish and sophistication to know how to dine properly. For links to tutorials on place settings, utensils and fine dining, go to www.ydkWydk.com.

• Utensils are placed in the anticipated order of use from the outside in. Salad fork to the outside of dinner fork and soup spoon to the outside of the dinner knife.

• Since most people are right handed, drinking glasses are on the right.

• Forks on the left. Smaller salad fork outside of the larger dinner fork.

• Knives and spoons on the right (most people are right handed and you cut with the right hand). Soup spoon to the outside.

• Dinner plate in the middle, bread plate to the left.

• Salad plate to the left.

• Dessert spoon and fork horizontal above the dinner plate.

• Napkin is usually on the plate, under the forks or sometimes in your glass.

• If you cannot remember whose bread plate is whose as the meal begins, put both hands out in front of you and touch your index finger to your thumb to form a circle and with your other fingers straight up you will form a "b" for bread with your left hand and a "d" for drink with your right hand. This tells you which bread plate and drinking glass is yours.

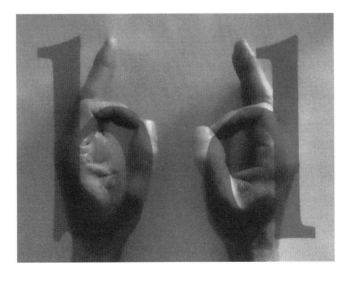

Using your Utensils

There are two basic styles of using your eating utensils, the American and European.

• American Style: Right hand holds the knife, left hand the fork. Object to be cut is in the center of the plate, the fork is used to stabilize the food with face down and curve up. Knife is used in a slow back and forth motion until object is cut. Then knife is placed at top of plate. Switch fork from left to right hand and pick up food to eat.

• Never place a used utensil back on the table; it should be placed on your plate.

• Always use your knife with control.

• If you drop your knife or fork in a fine restaurant, do not bend over and get it. Ask the server to replace it.

• When you are done eating, the fork and knife are placed together at the 4 o'clock position.

• The European or Continental style is similar to the American when cutting food but after cutting the piece, instead of switching the fork to the right hand, fork remains in the left hand and knife remains in the right hand. The food object brought to the mouth with the left hand. When done eating the knife is placed at the 4 o'clock position and the fork at the 8 o'clock position.

Tipping

Tipping is a part of our society and in some cases, a key portion of the server's income. If service is poor then the tip is reduced; if excellent, the tip should be generous. Bear in mind, service professions are demanding and often thankless; err towards generosity.

- Tipping is individual and changes with each situation.

- Base your tip in the <u>pre-tax</u> amount of the bill, not the total.

- Be discreet and avoid flashing cash or talking about your tip.

- In restaurants, tip 15-20% of the pre-tax bill depending on the service, the area and the time spent eating. If service is extremely poor, tip 8% (most restaurants report 8% tips for wait staff to the IRS; anything less costs the wait staff). Just make the point that you are unhappy with the service.

- You are under no obligation to give money to tip jars on countertops if you have not been provided table service by a waiter or waitress.

- At buffet or self service restaurants, 10% tip is adequate.

- If gratuity has already been added (usually 15-18%), add additional tip only if service was exceptional.

- If your meal was lengthy, more than 8 guests, or your meal was especially light during a busy time, then additional tip may be indicated.

- Bartenders should be tipped 15-20% if you are sitting at the bar for a while or you have been given exceptional service. Tip $1-2 per drink if you are not at the bar or waiting for a table at the restaurant. If you are in a crowded establishment, tip well for your first drink and talk directly to the bartender. Next time, your service should be excellent.

- Valet parking attendants are tipped $1-2 when the car is returned to you, not when you arrive.

- Luggage handlers and bellhops $1-2 per bag.

- Doorman $1-4.

- Taxi cab drivers 15% of fare.

- Housekeeping staff $2-5 per night depending on the quality of hotel.

- Concierge $5-10 per special event.

- Hairdresser 15-20%.

- Pizza or take out food delivery person 10%.

Money 101

Money cannot buy happiness. However, financial success eases life's hardships and significantly decreases stress. There are two keys to accumulating wealth: making money and keeping the money you've made. An understanding of economics, business and personal finance is essential and will reap substantial rewards over a lifetime. The fundamentals and pitfalls to avoid:

Principles

Interest - Interest is the price paid on the principal of any loan, be it a student loan, home loan, car loan, appliance purchase or credit card balance. Conversely, it is the also the return received from savings accounts, CDs and other financial investments. It is usually expressed as a percentage/year.

Compound Interest - With time, interest that accrues from an investment, loan or debt is added to the principal. From then on, interest is paid or charged on that interest. This is the power of long term investment, and the penalty for not paying debt off quickly.

Inflation - A measure of the rising cost of goods/services in an economy over time. US inflation averages about 3% since 1914. Inflation causes the purchasing power of your dollar to gradually decrease every year.

True Cost - This pertains to calculating the total, long term cost of any purchase but is commonly used for homes, cars, boats, toys and other large purchases which are paid for in installments. A common sales trick is to make the monthly payment low in an attempt to disguise the total cost. Take time and run all the numbers before making a decision. Example: A car loan of $25,000 at 5% interest for 5 years has a monthly payment of $472 and a total cost of $28,307.

Depreciation - The decrease in value of an item over time and use. This applies to nearly everything. Consider in making any purchase.

Money Smart Financial Education Program

http://www.fdic.gov/consumers/consumer/moneysmart/index.html

Provided by the FDIC, this is an in depth and unbiased course on money management in CD format and online. Excellent information and free.

Practices

Neither a borrower nor a lender be,
For loan oft loses both itself and friend,
And borrowing dulls the edge of husbandry.

<u>Hamlet</u>, William Shakespeare

Establish and Maintain a Budget - Sounds numbingly dull but a realistic budget pays off. Determine your needs, wants and an occasional splurge. Add monthly expenses to estimate your outflow. Eating out, clubbing and impulse buying adds up fast. Analyze both your financial situation and your temperament/personality and set a budget that you can adhere to.

Disciplined Spending - Impulse buying is a problem for any budget, especially with expensive items that you can't afford. Develop a ritual of delay: take 48 hours, research the cost, need and shop alternatives before committing to the purchase. The deal will still be there.

Never Loan Money - Other than cab fare or small change, avoid loans to friends, coworkers or relatives. Consider such loans as gifts. You have no way to assess collateral or credit risk and have no legal recourse. Politely refer them to your bank. If a bank with lawyers and access to credit data and the ability to lien collateral will not loan to them, you certainly shouldn't.

Always Get It In Writing - This means any agreement, repair or job estimate, promise, important discussion, etc. An email or signed fax will help if a signed contract is not possible. Do <u>not</u> be timid or embarrassed to expect an agreement to be put in writing; verbal or 'handshake' deals are completely worthless. If the other party refuses, this is a red flag. Avoid them and move on.

Credit Cards - Credit cards have two valid uses: cashless convenience and consumer protection for purchases. They should never be used as a way to borrow money, short or long term. This mistake will cost you dearly, can ruin your credit score, and is the #1 cause of bankruptcy in young adults. It is a good policy to pay off all credit card debt completely each month because interest rates on credit cards are typically high. This will save you money and help you control and budget your spending. If you only pay the 'minimal payment' required each month, you are in essence using the credit card as a long term loan, at rates of as much as 22 % per year. Make it a priority to pay the balance in full every month.

Study Method

Textbook Studies

Read the assigned textbook chapters before class. The professor assumes that the class has read the assigned chapter, so the lecture will make more sense if you have read the text. You will retain more and understand more. Furthermore, if you don't read the chapter before class, you will have two chapters to read before the next class. Stay ahead of the class work. Don't get behind.

Take comprehensive notes on the chapter or section. Reading the material is important, but you also need to remember it for the test. By taking notes you condense the important parts, making it easier for you later when you are studying for the test. And the act of writing the notes is a mnemonic device. You retain much more by converting the ideas in the book into notes and writing them down than by just reading and highlighting. You also have to select what is important enough to write in your notes, which helps you understand and remember the information.

Lectures

Go to class and take extensive lecture notes. Obviously the lecture is important; moreover the lecture is what the professor thinks is important and therefore is likely to be on the exam. Again, if you have done the reading, the lecture will make more sense and you can ask and answer questions in class. If you have an intelligent question, don't be afraid to ask it.

Review

This is the beginning of preparation for the test, and will save time when you get closer to exams. You will need all the time you can get when midterms and finals hit. Read the chapter again with the lecture in mind and add to your notes as needed. Focus on what the professor covered in lecture. Update textbook notes if the professor's lecture focused on areas of the chapter that you didn't think were important the first time you read it.

Studying for the Test

Before the test, read your two sets of notes (chapter + lecture), and the textbook as needed. Then, write a third set of notes, which is a compilation of the two. Use this summary to study for the test. Again, the act of writing the notes is a mnemonic device. You retain much more by gathering the ideas in the notes into a synopsis and writing it down than by just reading the notes.

Another option is to put key points on index flash cards. Put a question on one side and the answer on the other (or a vocabulary term on one side and the definition on the other). With flash cards you can carry them around and go through them as you have down time throughout the day. Go through the deck of flashcards, separate the cards you get right from the ones you get wrong, and go through the wrong deck again. Repeat.

Excellent grades and scores are attainable. The harder a subject is for you, the more time you have to spend on the class, but you can get an A in any class. You can get an A in every class. After the first semester you should have a better idea of how much you will have to study to get A's, and so you can amend this study method. The better you are in the subject, the less time you will need to spend on the class. But in the first semester, you should do the entire method for every class. Time is never wasted in study.

Don't Get Behind

You are going to have a lot of homework, so don't put it off. Get it done first. In your first semester you may not know how long homework takes and how to allot your time. Start homework early and have free time after, rather than free time first and run out of time for study. If you are caught up, you will enjoy your free time more. In fact, if you are caught up, try reading ahead. Being on top of it feels good. Success breeds success.

Get Help

If you are having trouble with a class, ask for help. Ask your teacher, your advisor, your parents, your friends. Don't get behind.

FINAL THOUGHTS

"Life is a sum of all your choices."

Albert Camus   1913-1960

Eight Healthy Habits To Start Today

in·er·tia *noun* : a term in physics, relating to matter, stating that a body at rest tends to stay at rest, and a body in motion tends to stay in motion.

Inertia affects human behavior as well as matter. Change is not easy; old habits die hard. But the truth is that humans can change. We as a species are changing and evolving, and as individuals we can evolve as well. We must. In the Stone Age, life was stagnant for generations, and human adaptation was minimal. In the 21st century, knowledge advances so rapidly that change is essential. The most successful humans will be the ones who can and do change.

Neurophysiology studies have shown that the human mind can change and adapt, but that neural reprogramming takes two or three weeks. Be patient, allow your brain pathways to change. Integrate these eight, positive behaviors into your routine to enhance your health and well being.

1. Start taking a quality daily multivitamin and mineral supplement.

2. Start a daily 30 minute exercise routine. Begin with walking and progress.

3. Start reading the nutritional label and ingredient list on every food you buy. Avoid foods with bad fats, high sodium, high sugar and HFCS.

4. Replace your butter, margarine and cooking oils with canola oil and canola oil margarine.

5. Choose foods close to the farm such as fresh fruits, vegetables and whole grains. Avoid processed foods.

6. Avoid fried foods, HFCS and red meat.

7. Drink alcohol in moderation or not at all. Excessive drinking is destructive in every aspect of life: health, professional and social.

8. Improve your hand washing technique and frequency. Carry hand sanitizer in your car, briefcase or purse. Stop touching your face, nose, mouth and eyes with dirty hands.

Core Life Philosophy

Your body is a temple. Be selfish about your health and take care of yourself first and foremost. Eat the right food, get sleep and exercise often. Don't follow the fools: resist peer pressure to binge drink or use drugs.

Seek, expect and demand excellence and integrity from those close to you. You <u>will</u> be judged by the quality and character of your friends. There is guilt by association; if you travel with thieves, how can honest men know that you are not a thief? High quality companions elevate you, teach you and inspire you. Troubled individuals add nothing and will invariably, eventually drag you down.

Luck favors the always prepared. Adopt the philosophy: "Prepare for the worse but expect the best." Life is unpredictable and no one can prepare for everything, but there are many simple, daily practices that, once integrated into your lifestyle, will help keep you healthy, safe and out of danger.

Study. Your college years determine your direction and success for the next forty years. Have fun and meet new people but take your studies seriously. Learn all you can, find what you enjoy doing and excel at it. Time and energy invested now will pay windfall dividends in later life.

Be a traveler. Take every opportunity to broaden your horizons. Study abroad, work in new places and explore the USA. Travel takes you out of your comfort zone, introduces you to new cultures and expands your perspectives.

Show respect and courtesy to everyone you encounter. It is just so much easier than conflict, and diminishes your internal stress and anger. Contribute to your community. Believe in karma and practice living well.

Get out, enjoy life and endeavor to never stop learning.

References and Resources

Health

The Mayo Clinic
www.mayoclinic.com

WebMD
www.webMD.com

Center for Science in the Public Interest
www.cspinet.org

US Food and Drug Administration
www.fda.gov

American Cancer Society
www.cancer.org

American Dental Association
www.ada.org

The American Heart Association
www.americanheart.org and http://handsonlycpr.org

The World Health Organization
www.WHO.int

American Lung Association
www.lungusa.org

Beers, M.H. MD. Editor-in-Chief. The Merck Manual of Medical Information, New York, Simon & Schuster, Inc.2003.

American Medical Association. The American Medical Association Family Medical Guide, 4th Edition, Hoboken, NJ. Wiley. 2004.

American Red Cross. First Aid/CPR/AED for Schools and the Community. Yardly, PA. Stay Well Publications. 2006.

Kramer SA. "Effect of Povidone-iodine on wound healing: a review." J Vasc Nurs. 1999 Mar;17(1):17-23

Nutrition

US Department of Agriculture

www.mypyramid.gov

US Food and Drug Administration

www.fda.gov

US Food Safety

www.foodsafety.gov

Centers for Disease Control and Prevention

www.cdc.gov

Bocarsly, Powell, Avena, Hoebel. "High-fructose corn syrup causes characteristic of obesity in rats: Increased body weight, body fat and triglyceride levels." Pharmacology Biochemistry and Behavior, 2010; DOI: 10.1016/j.pbb.2010.02.012.

Elliot, SE et al. "Fructose, weight gain, and the insulin resistance syndrome." American Journal of Clinical Nutrition, Vol. 76, No. 5, 911-922, November 2002 .

Bray GA, Nielsen SJ, Popkin BM. "Consumption of high-fructose corn syrup may play a role in the epidemic of obesity." Am J Clin Nutr Vol.79, No 4, 537-543, April 2004.

Exercise

American College of Sports Medicine

www.acsm.org

A Discovery Communications website

www.howstuffworks.com

A New York Times Company website

www.about.com

Men's Health Magazine

www.menshealth.com

Safety

Underwriters Laboratories

www.ul.com

Kidde Fire Fighting

www.kidde-fire.com

Federal Bureau of Investigation

www.fbi.gov

The Federal Government Source for Women's Health Information

www.womenshealth.gov

The Brady Campaign to Prevent Gun Violence

www.bradycampaign.org

Federal Premium Ammunition

www.federalpremium.com

277

Arizona Department of Public Safety

www.azdps.gov

National Criminal Justice Reference Service, US Department of Justice

http://www.ncjrs.gov/App/Publications/abstract.aspx?ID=97119

Fieldbook: The BSA's Manual of Advanced Skills for Outdoor Travel, Adventure and Caring for the Land, 4th Edition. Irving, Tx. Boy Scouts of America. 2004.

Travel

Tripadvisor

www.tripadvisor.com

Frommer's Travel Guide, for travel destination information

www.frommers.com

Fodors's Travel Guide, for travel destination information

www.fodors.com

Transportation Security Administration

www.tsa.gov

American Automobile Association

www.aaa.com

Detective Kevin Coffey, Travel Safety Expert

www.kevincoffee.com

Peter Greenberg, Worldwide Travel News and Tips

www.petergreenberg.com

Recreational Equipment Inc (REI), for outdoor advice

www.rei.com/expertadvice

Rick Steves, Travel expert - European travel

www.ricksteves.com

Greenberg, P. The Travel Detective. New York, Villard Books, 2001.

Wise, M. MD, The Travel Doctor. Buffalo, NY. Firefly Books, 2002.

Fieldbook: The BSA's Manual of Advanced Skills for Outdoor Travel, Adventure and Caring for the Land, 4th Edition. Irving, Tx. Boy Scouts of America. 2004.

Auto

American Automobile Association

www.aaa.com

AAA Foundation for Traffic Safety

www.aaafoundation.org

Edmunds Car Review and Pricing

www.edmunds.com

Road and Travel Magazine

www.roadandtravel.com

Mothers Against Drunk Driving

www.MADD.org

National Highway Traffic Safety Administration

www.nhtsa.dot.gov

Kelley Blue Book Car Values

www.kbb.com

Consumer Reports

www.consumerreports.org

Prevent Blindness America

www.preventblindness.org

Keys to Success

Emily Post Etiquette

www.emilypost.com

Consumers Reports

www.consumerreports.org

Greener Choices, the green website for eco-living

www.greenerchoices.org

Clorox Cleaning Products

www.clorox.com

Peggy Post. Emily Post's Etiquette 7th Edition. William Morrow, 2004.

The Editors of Consumers Reports with Edward Kippel. How to Clean Practically Anything, Fourth Edition, Yonkers NY, Consumer Reports Books, 1996.

Index

About the Authors

Philip Bhaskar, DMD

Dr. Philip Bhaskar attended the University of Florida and graduated with a Bachelor's Degree in Chemistry. He received his DMD degree from the University of Florida College of Dentistry. Dr. Bhaskar completed a General Practice Residency at the UCLA-Wadsworth VA Medical Center, his Oral and Maxillofacial Surgery Residency at the University of Florida and a Fellowship in Oral and Maxillofacial Surgery at the University of Florida. Dr Bhaskar is Board Certified by the American Board of Oral and Maxillofacial Surgery and is a Fellow of the American Association of Oral and Maxillofacial Surgeons.

William Bhaskar, MD

Dr. William Bhaskar attended the University of Illinois, Urbana-Champaign and the University of Colorado, graduating with a Bachelor's of Science degree in Biology. He studied as a graduate student at Georgetown University Medical School, and was a medical researcher at the University of Texas Medical School in San Antonio. He received his MD from the University of Texas Medical Branch, Galveston and did his General Surgery training at the Phoenix Integrated Surgical Residency in Arizona. Plastic Surgery residency was completed at the University of California, Davis Medical Center. Dr. Bhaskar is Board Certified by the American Board of Plastic Surgery.

2686386R00167

Made in the USA
San Bernardino, CA
23 May 2013